... ... Bryan, herself an eminent paediatrician and ... ...< specialist, shows that we are all more than the product of our genes. Her indomitable spirit and expansive humanity make this an uplifting and optimistic account; I was left in no doubt that I had just spent time with a truly remarkable woman.'

Baroness Helena Kennedy QC,
Chair of the Human Genetics Commission

'Whether you are caring for someone with cancer or dealing with it yourself, the thought inevitably goes through your mind – if I knew more, could I do more? Elizabeth Bryan provides an immensely valuable triple perspective as a carer, a patient and a doctor, which makes essential reading for anyone facing the challenge of cancer in whatever form. This book can be read as a story of human courage, a source of advice and information or a fascinating contribution to the implications of genetic testing.'

Lindsay Nicholson, author of *Living on the Seabed*

'Dr bryan's personal strength, honesty and compassion wiil make it a helpful and inspiring story for others . . . This is a book that we would recommend to everyone involved in the clinical management and counselling about familiar cancer and those who want to understand what it is realy like to live with a family history of cancer.'

Human Fertility

'This lucid, wise and courageous book makes an invaluable and original contribution to the current spiritual debate. At a time when it is all too easy to push unwelcome reality to the periphery of our consciousness, Elizabeth Bryan shows that it is possible to live in the shadow of death with grace, compassion and humour. Without a trace of self-pity, she reminds us that life can only be fully savoured if we learn to accept our mortality. After reading her story, death loses much of its terror.'

Karen Armstrong, author of *A History of God*

'*Singing the Life* is a unique insight into the heart of a family living with inherited cancer. Its eloquence and honesty are inspiring. Those in the shadow of cancer should read it. Those who counsel people at genetic risk must read it.'

ics,
sity

For
Max, Liz, Ben and Catherine

And to the memory of
Alice

Singing the Life

*The story of a family in
the shadow of cancer*

ELIZABETH BRYAN MD FRCP FRCPCH

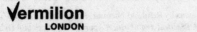
Vermilion
LONDON

1 3 5 7 9 10 8 6 4 2

First published in 2007 by Vermilion, an imprint of Ebury Publishing
This edition published by Vermilion in 2008

Ebury Publishing is a Random House Group company

Copyright © Elizabeth Bryan 2007

Elizabeth Bryan has asserted her right to be identified as the author of this Work
in accordance with the Copyright, Designs and Patents Act 1988.

The Random House Group Limited Reg. No. 954009

Addresses for companies within the Random House Group can be found at
www.rbooks.co.uk

A CIP catalogue record for this book is available from the British Library

The Random House Group Limited supports The Forest Stewardship
Council (FSC), the leading international forest certification organisation.
All our titles that are printed on Greenpeace approved FSC certified paper
carry the FSC logo. Our paper procurement policy can be found at
www.rbooks.co.uk/environment

Printed in the UK by CPI Cox & Wyman, Reading, RG1 8EX

ISBN 9780091917166

Copies are available at special rates for bulk orders. Contact the sales
development team on 020 7840 8487 or visit www.booksforpromotions.co.uk
for more information.

To buy books by your favourite authors and register for offers, visit
www.rbooks.co.uk

The publishers have made every reasonable effort to contact the copyright owners
of the extracts reproduced in this book. In the few cases where they have been
unsuccessful they invite copyright holders to contact them direct and corrections
can be made in reprints.

Extracts from *Anam Cara* by John O'Donohue, *It's Not Like That Actually* by Kate
Carr and *C: Because Cowards Get Cancer Too* by John Diamond have been
reproduced by permission of The Random House Group Ltd.

Prayers by Reinhold Niebuhr, Margaret Torrie, and Thomas Nerton, as quoted in
A Practical and Spiritual Approach to Death and Dying by Bill Kirkpatrick, have
been reproduced with kind permission by Darton, Longman and Todd.

Contents

Prologue

I sing the life that is born in all of us,
Ours to use the best way we can.
I sing the death that is yet in store for us
Linking back to the place we began.

Jane Mayers, 1987

IN JUNE 2005 I was diagnosed with a life-threatening cancer of
the pancreas, which could possibly be due to the same
abnormality in the gene that had caused the ovarian cancer and
death of my sister Bunny and two episodes of breast cancer in
my other sister Felicity, as well as the death of at least five of our
other relatives and possibly many more. Our father had been a
carrier of the BRCA1 cancer gene and we had inherited this
from him. As BRCA1 is a dominant gene, each of my three
nieces and two nephews had a 50/50 chance of being similarly
affected.

During my convalescence from extensive surgery and the
subsequent six months of chemotherapy, I have had many
hours to reflect on what this inherited cancer has meant. Meant
to me personally, to us as a family and to future generations
who must face choices, with the ethical and psychological

dilemmas they carry, some of which were not even available to my sisters and me when we first discovered we could be carrying BRCA1.

I have also thought about how illness and bereavement has affected each of us in different ways, and have reflected, perhaps most of all, on how they have brought a deeper and stronger aspect to relationships both within our family and among our wide circle of friends.

Although I am a doctor, cancer is not my own area of expertise. Yet, as a paediatrician who has specialised in twins and triplets for over 30 years, I have inevitably become interested in genetics, to which twin studies make such a contribution. And, unavoidably, bereavement counselling has always been part of my work because multiple birth infants tend to be especially vulnerable both during pregnancy and the first few days after they are born.

So now, on the other side of the fence, I have also been able to think about being a patient, and one whose life is threatened. I have come to regret how much better a doctor I might have been, had I been at the receiving end of medical care earlier in my career. In the past 18 months I have learnt as many lessons from sometimes unwittingly insensitive doctors and nurses as from many others whose patience, encouragement and quiet humour have sustained me through dark times.

It is these experiences, reflections and lessons that I shall try to share in this book.

One thing that this last year has done for me is to make it easier to admit to myself what I truly feel. Writing this book has helped me explore these feelings further, some of which I never knew I had until I started putting them on paper. Some are embarrassing, even shaming. Many I have shared with very few others.

If I survive to see this book published, I could come to regret being so open. I hope not. But even if I do, my fervent hope will remain that *Singing the Life* may add to the understanding of inherited cancers and perhaps other diseases and, most of all, that it may help and comfort some fellow travellers, their relatives, friends or carers, without causing undue distress to those closest and dearest to me.

Part One
The Background

I

A Family History of Cancer

I HAVE HAD three bolts from the blue that have changed my life. One in 1948 at the age of six, one in 1973 and then, the third, in 2005 when I developed cancer.

My first bolt I remember mostly through the memories of my parents. Having watched a film about African children in hospital, I decided to be a children's doctor. Thereafter I never wavered. When doubt over exams loomed, I would sometimes weaken in my medical ambition, but never in my wish to work with children.

I always loved being with children. As a teenager, I would be called upon to arrange children's parties, or to conduct the under fives class at pony club. Later, an unmarried and childless paediatrician was the obvious choice for godparent, and over the years I acquired 14 godchildren, all of whom have given me enormous pleasure. For several years I held godchildren's camps in the orchard of my little cottage on the North York Moors. It is touching how many of them still remember the fishing expeditions to Whitby, 'mystery tours' over the moors, the leaking tents and damp barbecues.

They would teasingly suggest potential husbands for me and

plan their bridesmaids' dresses. We talked of the children I would have, of the help they would give when they eventually arrived. As it turned out it is I who enjoy my godchildren's own children. I have 16 grand-godchildren and more are due this year. To my sadness I have never had any children of my own.

The second bolt hit on a cold night in March 1973 at Hammersmith Hospital. I was the junior paediatrician 'on call'. Twins were about to be delivered. I do not know who was the more surprised, the mother or me, as the two baby boys emerged. One was a bouncing, bright red six-pounder and the other pale and wizened, weighing little more than three pounds. This was my first experience of twin–twin transfusion syndrome, where during the pregnancy one baby transfuses blood, and hence most of the food supply, into the other one. I decided to find out more.

The quest marked the beginning not only of a two-year research project on the placenta in a twin pregnancy but of my preoccupation ever since with the nature and nurture of multiple births and their families. A few minutes in the delivery ward had given birth to one pair of twins and a life's work.

The third bolt should have arrived in 1975 but its full impact did not hit me for another 30 years. For in February of that year I received what should have struck me as a highly significant letter from Dr Nancy Maguire, one of my father's eight first cousins from his mother's side of the family. She wrote:

I am writing this circular letter with its enclosures, to the medical members of the family. As you will see from the enclosed family tree there is already a 50 per cent incidence of ovarian cancer diagnosed in our family on the Hall side in two generations. Both I and Farquhar Macrae [another of my father's first cousins] feel that it is vital that the girls of the next generation to us are fully informed and can discuss this family case history with their gynaecologists.

Before this I had no idea that cancer was common in our family. Nancy Maguire's letter went on to discuss the family tree and possible source of the cancer, pointing out that my grandmother, Sylvie, and my grandmother's half-sister, my great-aunt, had both died of ovarian cancer as had Nancy's own sister and her first cousin, my aunt Sylvia. Another cousin Margaret, née Macrae, had been successfully treated for the same cancer by radiotherapy.

She enclosed pathology reports from various members of the family showing that all had the same type of cancer of the ovary, an adenocarcinoma. She also pointed out that the age when the cancer appeared was falling. The two cases in my grandmother's generation were both in their sixties, in Nancy's generation two had been in their early fifties and one was 47. Of those afflicted, not all had had children and for four out of five the cancer had had a rapid course with none surviving more than two years.

She continued:

However the question arises as to whether it is male transmitted. This question is very important for Paul Bryan's daughters [myself, Felicity and Bunny], Farquhar Macrae's daughters and Norman Macrae's daughter. . . My personal feeling is that to be on the safe side, one has to assume the possibility of male

transmission, at least to the extent of careful specialist gynae-
cological monitoring.

Nancy said that, in view of the family history, which meant that
she herself had a 50/50 chance of inheriting the cancer gene she
had recently had a hysterectomy with both ovaries removed and
was encouraging her younger sister to do the same. She went on:

> I am most thankful that I had an understanding of the
> implications of the family history in this very silent disease, and
> was in the hands of a gynaecologist who took it seriously and was
> prepared to take preventive action.
>
> I have written this letter to alert some of the more far-flung
> members of the family who may not be aware of the details of
> this medical family tree, so that they can contact all the Hall
> descended female cousins they know of who come into this 'at
> risk' category, so that they can present the facts to their
> gynaecologists for evaluation and careful monitoring.

Although I have always been in touch with two of my aunts and
some of my own first cousins, there are other members of
the family I do not know nearly as well. Of my more distant
family, I knew very little indeed until I started research for this
book. At that point I had never met any of my father's first
cousins, nor any of their 13 children and 23 grandchildren.
This is a very different picture to the current Bryan
grandchildren with their close relationships to their cousins
and their aunts.

As with my own generation, my father's family was widely
scattered. He had been born, like many of his eight siblings, in

Japan, where my grandfather was a professor of English as well as a writer, poet and priest. After a childhood divided between Japan and England, the family spread out across the globe: two brothers and a sister ended up in Canada, another sister in Australia, while my father, one brother and one sister settled in England. My father did keep in regular, if infrequent, touch with all his siblings but made little effort to contact his wider family, most of whom he hadn't seen during my lifetime. His seven surviving first cousins were scattered between the UK, Canada, South Africa and South Korea. Whether my father would have kept in closer touch had he been brought up with the ease of international travel of this generation's children, I don't know. In fact, he didn't see his own parents between the ages of 14 and 21.

In 1954, when I was 12, we did have a grand reunion of many of the Bryan family at our home in Yorkshire when four families reunited and nine young cousins met, some for the first time. This was one of the only two times that I met my Canadian aunt Sylvia Wevill. Not surprisingly her death in Canada at 54 and that, many years earlier, of my 67-year-old paternal grandmother, Sylvie, when I was three and whom I had never known, had little impact on me. I later learnt that they had both died of some kind of cancer.

Two months after receiving Nancy Maguire's letter, I received a letter from South Africa from Farquhar Macrae who had been a medical missionary in China for 19 years and then in South Africa, before becoming a GP there. In his letter he said:

Under the circumstances I am sure you will agree that Nancy was very wise to have a prophylactic [preventive] operation (and Heather [her sister] should have the same). Hilary Wevill [my first cousin] with a mother and grandmother affected she, too, should have an oophorectomy [removal of ovaries]. I am going to write accordingly though ethically and personally it smells of interference!

You will have realised that there is no proof from our family tree so far as to whether this cancer can be transmitted through the male – which would affect you and your sisters, my daughters and my brother's daughter.

He went on to say that he had discussed it with a competent geneticist who thought that it was inherently unlikely that transmission could be through the male.

Farquhar continued with a description of eight generations of our family tree and the likely source of the cancer gene. He commented that our cancer was unusual in so far being limited to the ovaries. In several reports of other families with inherited cancer, cancers of the breast as well as the ovary occurred within the same family.

At the time that Nancy's and Farquhar's letters arrived I was 33, unmarried and a junior paediatrician. I replied courteously but without much interest or enthusiasm. I created a file in my filing cabinet called Family Ovarian Cancer and forgot about it for several years. Indeed, until I started research for this book, I had completely forgotten how much detailed information I had been sent.

Looking back on it I am amazed and shocked by my reaction, or lack of it. Here were two cousins, whom I didn't even know, taking enormous trouble to provide us with warnings and relevant information about life-threatening but potentially avoidable dangers to our family, dangers that were no longer going to affect them personally. They had taken it upon themselves to apprise us fully of the risks not just to us but for future generations.

Had I been just too preoccupied by my own very full and exciting life? How did I manage to so effectively sweep all this under the carpet?

By birth and upbringing I am an optimist, like my mother. So was my father who, despite some tragic bereavements, always claimed that his life had been 'dogged by good luck'. His two main careers, the army and politics, came to him by chance. Out of 30 officers in his battalion who landed in Algeria he was the only one still in action there 12 months later. His luck persisted on the golf course: as a mediocre golfer he hit two holes in one in one round on the internationally renowned Ganton golf course, and hence got an entry in the *Guiness Book of Records*.

My parents had married in June 1939, just 10 weeks before the outbreak of World War Two. My father joined the Queen's Own Royal West Kent Regiment as a private. Because of the high casualty rate and his own leadership abilities he had a meteoric rise over four years from private to lieutenant colonel, winning a DSO (Distinguished Service Order) and an MC (Military Cross) along the way.

He returned from the war as a jobless hero, but was invited to join his father-in-law, my grandfather, running the family clothing company of JB Hoyle, in Hebden Bridge in the West Riding of Yorkshire. This never became a source of great excitement for him or of free fashion for his daughters. Its main lines were corduroy dungarees and boiler suits. Furthermore tan, drab and mouse are more fashionable colours now than they would have been then. Similarly the two fashion lines, the 'armaclad' and the more sophisticated 'smartaclad', did not have an immediate appeal.

My younger sister Felicity arrived just after the end of the war, when I was three. Three years later, in 1948, my youngest sister Bunny completed the family. And a happy family we were. My mother had trained as a physiotherapist but after the war enthusiastically devoted her energies to being a full-time mother.

We lived in a cottage outside Halifax, across the field from our grandparents' much larger house, which with its woods and lawns was an ideal place for entertaining friends, for games, picnics and hide and seek. A large pond was the focus for swimming parties or rides in my rowing boat, the 'Libby-loo', an eighth birthday present from my grandfather.

As children we were close, mainly perhaps because our parents were committed to family life and shared many of our activities. Serious arguments or disagreements were discouraged, not always easily as our personalities were very different. Felicity enjoyed baiting an easily provoked younger sister. I was the classic eldest child: large for my age, bossy, anxious, over-conscientious and a typical, not outstanding, schoolgirl. Felicity was the opposite: enviably petite, vague, uncompetitive, artistic and musical. She saw no point in school and was usually late for it.

Our age difference was such that at both junior and senior schools I was at the top when she was at the bottom. Discipline was not for her and she delighted in ensuring that her young friends quickly lost any respect for my prefectorial authority. This was the time when Felicity and I had our least good relationship.

Bunny, teasingly nicknamed 'buttercup fairy', loved her food, was extremely determined and strove to keep up with her elder sisters. To the distress of my peace-loving mother, she would have ferocious temper tantrums when she failed. By four, Bunny would be seen and heard bossily trying to organise her seven-year-old sister. She was already the same height and considerably heavier.

It is fascinating to see some of these traits in their children but no longer in either of my sisters. They both changed a lot over the years. Unfortunately they would probably say I have changed much less. Felicity is now renowned for her energy, productivity and organising skills, whereas Bunny became the most peaceful and reflective of the three of us with little regard for time, and none for aggression or conflict.

With such different personalities, our life paths might well have diverged had not family circumstances continued to unite us. We all adored my mother and, in our teenage years, were firmly united in our efforts to sustain her through her long depressive illness. Similarly, during my father's widowhood and the many family crises that came later, the one unquestionable bonus was our being drawn closer. This now seems to be happening to the next generation, who have already had to face a number of tragedies together.

Although by 1949 my father was happily settled in Halifax, he found business life tame after the front lines of battle. Then, out of the blue, he was asked to fight as the Conservative candidate in a parliamentary by-election in the local Sowerby constituency. He had no previous experience or particular interest in politics but my mother was always keen on adventure and encouraged him by saying, 'It will be more fun than not.'

He lost three parliamentary elections in Sowerby but his enthusiasm had been fired and in 1955 he became the member for Howden, a large rural constituency on the Wolds of Yorkshire's East Riding. Here he remained for over 30 years, during this time becoming a minister and vice-chairman of his party.

It was three years earlier, in 1952, when I was 10, that my mother decided the family needed a change of scene. We moved to Park Farm, high on the edge of the North York Moors looking across the Vale of Pickering to the Wolds. Here we were introduced to a whole new and exciting life, which must have surprised our far more serious farming neighbours. Our Jersey cows were named after family members and the less aristocratic ones after friends. Deliciously rich and unhealthy butter took hours to make in the wooden churn; orphaned baby rabbits were nurtured in blanket boxes, sickly piglets in the bottom of the Aga.

In the summer we galloped our shaggy ponies along the forest's sandy tracks and in the winter were pulled along the same tracks by the Land Rover on our sledges or skis. There were other families on the farm so we became a formidable gang of seven children who encouraged each other in many a hair-raising exploit. Our mother was as thrilled as we were by this new life and welcomed a steady stream of visiting children, organising treasure hunts in the dale, bicycle rides over the moors, regular visits to an icy sea at Scarborough and fishing expeditions from Whitby.

Not only did we three children now have this new country

life but also, once my father had entered Parliament, the bonus of a family flat in London, a whole new world of friends. Throughout it all we enjoyed the unqualified love of two proud parents who were endlessly encouraging but not overprotective. Independence and adventure was expected sometimes at the expense of safety. From an early age one of us would be put in charge of the map reading for expeditions or, with dictionary in hand, the food shopping when we were lent an apartment in Paris.

At 10 I was driving a tractor with trailer laden with stooks of corn when it ran away with me. Keen that we should pass our driving tests soon after we turned 17, we were taught to drive on the forest tracks for many years before. As soon as legally allowed, I was charged with driving Felicity and Bunny and their ponies to pony club or to meets of the local hunt where my trailer-reversing efforts were often a hazard to other hunt followers. Only two months after my test I became the main driver over the mountain roads when my mother and I went off to Italy in our Morris Minor for three weeks.

Until I was 18 I doubt that I could have had a fuller or happier life. Then disaster struck. I was in my first year of medical school. My mother developed a profound depression that led on to phases of mania during which she became a completely different person. She had been widely loved. Now she could be arrogant, insensitive, irresponsible, even abusive, and wildly inconsistent.

The whole family suffered. I gave up a year's medical training to help out. It was hardest of all for Bunny who was only 12 at the time. Home was no longer a place of fun and laughter, but of sadness and anxiety. Her school holidays were often lonely, with home life sustained only by our grandmother who was by then living with us. I was often a poor substitute for parents unable to take Bunny out for the day from her boarding school in Kent. I loved my youngest sister and with our wide age gap had never had problems of conflict or competition. I enjoyed this premature parenting role but it was far from ideal for her and it inevitably gave us an unequal relationship. For Bunny this took many years to relinquish, at least until after the birth of her own children, and perhaps never entirely.

Occasionally we saw glimpses of the mother we remembered. Most of the time she was either profoundly depressed or manically destructive. Twice she made serious attempts to kill herself. Family life was entirely unpredictable. After eight agonising years, during a brief remission while holidaying with my father in Spain, she died, apparently peacefully, early one morning in the hotel swimming pool. It was a release and a relief. She had probably drowned during a dizzy spell caused by her medication. She would never have intentionally taken her life during one of the rare periods of happiness.

That was seven years before Nancy Maguire's letter about which I had done nothing. Was I worrying so much about the risks of inheriting my mother's bipolar disorder that I was unable to take on board the significance of a cancer that had not yet affected anyone to whom I was emotionally close, and still seemed remote? Unlike my nephews and nieces now, I had had no intimate experience of cancer. I had experienced the death of people close to me from accident, war, heart disease and suicide, but never from cancer.

Or had I just latched on to one geneticist's belief? The one who suggested that transmission through the father was unlikely and so I had unconsciously decided to ignore the various references to scientific papers on male transmission that Farquhar had provided for me? If men could not transmit the cancer gene, my sisters and I would be safe.

I should have known better. Even though knowledge of genetics was much more limited in the seventies it should still have been clear to me that the cancer appeared to be caused by a dominant gene and was therefore just as likely to be transmitted through male as female family members. Nor was I a stranger to medical research and how to survey the literature, even if it wasn't as easy then as now via the Internet. There were still the tomes of the *Index Medicus*, with which I was very familiar having completed my MD thesis on 'Placental Transfer of Immunoglobulins in Multiple Pregnancy' only a few years before.

In 1995 my sister Bunny died of cancer. Had my apathy, laziness, ignorance, denial, lack of interest, whatever it was, delayed the diagnosis of her illness, I would have undoubtedly felt responsible for her death. I don't know how I would have lived with that. Fortunately I had learnt much more about the gene before the first signs of Bunny's cancer had appeared and had given her and Felicity the relevant information and advice. So, more by luck than virtue, I did not have to bear that particularly dreadful guilt. This was no help to her, only to my conscience.

In 1982, seven years after the first letter, I had another from Farquhar Macrae in which he sent me a copy of a carefully researched talk he had given to the Eastern Province Branch of the Medical Association of South Africa titled 'Genetics and GPs'. In this he presented the medical history of our family in eight generations over 200 years. Inevitably the causes of death in the earlier generations were not always accurately known and some had died early in life before they would have had time to develop cancer. Even in the seventh generation two young girl cousins had died of infections. One young male in the sixth and another in the seventh had been killed in the First and Second World Wars respectively. Another male in the sixth generation had died young of diabetes, before treatment with insulin was available.

Nevertheless, what was clearly apparent in the later generations was the unusual frequency of other cancers *in addition* to the six cases of ovarian cancer. In the fifth generation my great-grandfather Hall was thought to have died of cancer of the stomach. In the seventh generation there were four other cases of cancer. Among the males there were two cases of cancer of the prostate, one of lung cancer and another of stomach cancer. In the eighth generation, my own, one of my first cousins had already died of a malignant melanoma.

In his talk Farquhar pointed out that a generation could be missed and the disease reoccur in a grandchild, as in the case of Marjorie Marsden. That was to say that a mother could carry the gene and, without getting cancer herself, hand it on to her daughter.

Despite all this information, I was not unduly perturbed, and certainly not preoccupied by this threat to our family. Felicity cannot remember it making any impact on her at all. As a doctor I felt obliged to act responsibly but did so with little enthusiasm. It is only now, talking to younger members of our family, that I realise that perhaps my slow response to the warnings was not unusual. Cancer and death are far from most young minds, thank goodness. There are so many much more immediate things to be interested in and indeed to worry about.

I wrote back to Farquhar:

> I am afraid I have been relatively complacent about it [our family cancer] as far as my sisters and I were concerned as I had been under the misapprehension that it was transmitted through the female only.
>
> Obviously we must now get expert genetic advice on the question of prophylactic oophorectomy. As I work at Queen Charlotte's and the Hammersmith Hospitals in London, I have access to the necessary expertise.
>
> As we are all three still childless we would obviously be reluctant to do anything yet... we [Ronald and I] are still hoping to have children although we have been unsuccessful so far. Felicity at 36 is currently pregnant with her first child and Bunny, aged 33, is unmarried.

In another letter later in 1982, Farquhar said that in the 200 members of our wider family he had managed to trace, there had been no known cases of breast cancer and no cases of ovarian cancer outside the Bryan, Marsden and Macrae families. Felicity's cancer in 2000 was, in fact, the first case of cancer in the breast in eight generations. Whether, had she not already had her ovaries removed, she would have developed ovarian cancer instead of breast cancer, we shall never know. In the same way, the previous absence of breast cancer in the family could perhaps be explained by the earlier deaths from ovarian cancer of other potential candidates.

But what is the picture in our family now? I had no idea

whether the more distant members of the family had continued to be afflicted by the BRCA1 cancer gene in the way we had. Since the letters from the two doctor cousins, Farquhar Macrae and Nancy Maguire, in the seventies and early eighties, I had had no further contact with them.

I have since managed to gather information on all 20 of my first and second cousins, their 45 children and, so far, 13 grandchildren. By 2006, none of them had suffered from cancer of either the ovary or breast. One had died of a malignant melanoma and another of cancer of the oesophagus. Three had had their wombs and ovaries removed as preventive measures.

In some of the families there have been no girls for several generations, which means that they do not know whether the cancer gene is still present in their branch of the family. In the family of one of my first cousins the gene has not had a chance to express itself in three successive generations. The first girl in that family was born in the fourth generation, in 2000, over 100 years after her last affected relative – a great-great-grandmother.

However, when the letters from Farquhar Macrae and Nancy Maguire arrived I was, perhaps not surprisingly, more preoccupied with the failures of my reproductive organs than whether they were harbouring a cancer. I had married Ronald Higgins in 1978 and we were eager to start a family. At 36 and 49 we realised there was no time to lose, but we were having trouble.

After having been a diplomat for 13 years in the UK and abroad, followed by several years on the staff of the *Observer*, Ronald left the newspaper in 1975 to write a book on global futures: *The Seventh Enemy: The Human Factor in the Global*

Crisis. This was published three years later, just before we were married.

Following an extraordinary response to a BBC television programme he made about the book, Ronald became increasingly involved with writing and lecturing about the various threats he saw, and foresaw, to the general global outlook. This work tied him less to London and it became feasible for us to move to our Herefordshire cottage on the Welsh border, which we both much preferred despite my job in London.

I had moved from York to join him in London and had a part-time appointment as a paediatrician at Queen Charlotte's and Chelsea Hospital in London. I would usually spend two or three days a week at the hospital and otherwise write from home or lecture in different parts of the country or overseas. My work was increasingly focusing on twins and triplets. Having helped to start the Twins and Multiple Births Association in 1978, I then, in 1988, gave up my general paediatric job to create and direct a new charity, the Multiple Births Foundation, aimed primarily at educating professional staff in the special problems faced by multiple birth children and their families.

Just after our first wedding anniversary, to our intense joy and relief, I became pregnant. We had never concealed the fact that we were trying hard and soon our family and friends were sharing our happiness. But 10 weeks into the pregnancy, I miscarried. Ronald and I wept together for the loss of our precious baby. I did not mourn the loss of motherhood. I assumed that if I had got pregnant once, I could do so again.

But as the months went by there was no sign of another pregnancy. Endless tests reassured both of us that we were functioning normally but disappointed us in that there was therefore nothing obvious to be done.

This was a difficult time, especially when my two younger sisters started producing children with apparent ease. Felicity, also now in her late thirties, had a daughter, Alice, and a son, Max, in quick succession followed three years later by another son, Ben. Bunny was married to Rob, a vicar, and had her two daughters, Lizzie and Catherine, in 1985 and 1988. I found this much harder than I had expected. Although my sisters were enormously sensitive to my feelings there was nothing they could do to reduce my envy or ease my longings as I watched the infinite pleasure the children gave to their parents and grandparents.

At times I became very angry. Why should I have been given such an instinctive love for children and apparent gifts for relating to them if I was not to be allowed any of my own?

I found the uncertainty, with the repeated disruption to our life that it caused, almost the hardest part to cope with. The problem of uncertainty was one I was again to find very difficult in the years to come, both with Ronald's cancer and even more with my own. At least later, the uncertainty no longer involved my work and career. But now, in mid-career, once we had agreed that children were our priority, I could not make any long-term plans about work.

As my fortieth birthday approached we were labelled as 'unexplained infertility'. We were told nothing more could be done. It was now just four years since the birth of the first baby, Louise Brown, from in vitro fertilization, IVF. The technique was still in its infancy and the success rate low. For those over 40 it was very low indeed. But after another set of tests my specialist agreed that I should have just one go, not least to convince ourselves that we had tried everything. I did not want to be haunted for ever afterwards by thoughts of 'if only'.

We had our one attempt. Only one egg fertilised. Before our one precious embryo was transferred to the womb I was allowed to look at it under the microscope: a few transparent, but live, cells. Never have I had a more heart-stopping sight and one in which such hope was invested. I have never forgotten it.

I returned to Herefordshire to wait. After the longest fortnight of my life, my period started. That was the end of our quest for a child.

Ronald and I briefly discussed adoption but for various reasons, including our ages – we were now 41 and 54 – we decided against it. Despite my longings for a child, I felt that if we were not able to have one ourselves, particularly when there was no obvious medical impediment, then our childlessness was somehow meant to be. However, despite this sort of rationalisation, I did not find this easy to accept at the time.

I still think about our own baby, the one who miscarried at 10 weeks. She – I somehow always felt she was a girl – would now be 26. I do sometimes resent the fact that in all the long saga of our infertility, people have forgotten, however understandably, about our one short-lived pregnancy and the baby it represented. But inevitably there have been compensations, as Ronald wrote in our book *Infertility: New Choices, New Dilemmas:*

> As the years have passed we have often talked about the family we never had, but about the benefits as well as the sadness of childlessness. When on the spur of the moment we decide to

spend an evening at the theatre or a weekend in the Welsh mountains we can mostly do just that. . . this is not the alleged selfishness of the childless: we could hardly have done more to generate the pitter-patter of tiny feet. Our task has changed: it has become one of making something good, both at work and play, out of the eventual failure of what had been our paramount hope.

2

BRCA1 and the Implications

BY 1990 I had decided to have regular ultrasound screening of my ovaries with a view to having my ovaries removed in the relatively near future. I discussed the plan with Felicity and Bunny and they agreed that screening was a good idea. But Felicity certainly does not remember thinking of having her ovaries removed at any point soon. As non-medical people, she and Bunny showed what to me seemed comparatively little interest.

Of course they were busy – Felicity juggling her job with three small children and Bunny working in Rob's parish and looking after two little daughters. Felicity got round to having the scan in the spring. But Bunny, taken up with other priorities, did not have it done till July 1991. Both were told there was no sign of cancer, though Felicity's specialist stressed that no scan was foolproof.

In April 1991, I received an unexpected letter from a research assistant at the recently established Cancer Research Campaign Genetics Research Group in Cambridge, where a register was being set up of families who appeared to have a hereditary form of ovarian cancer 'in order to do genetic linkage studies and also to coordinate and evaluate appropriate screening'. One of my cousins, already on the register, had given my name.

This group has now evolved into the UK Familial Ovarian Cancer Register (FOCR), and by 2006 the register had grown to include nearly 400 families with nearly 1,400 women taking part: the largest set of well-documented ovarian cancer families in the world. The main research aims of the group are to identify genes that increase the risk of ovarian cancer and to quantify cancer risks associated with a family history of ovarian cancer.

Some of the studies are carried out in collaboration with researchers from around the world. Details of medical and family history are being collected from families with two or more first- or second-degree relatives[1] on the same side of the family with ovarian cancer of a specific type. Blood samples are also collected from those happy to provide them.

It was 1991 and according to the state of knowledge at that time it appeared that about 1 or 2 per cent of all cases of ovarian cancer were due to a family gene and that the inheritance was an autosomal dominant pattern, which means that each child of a gene carrier had a 50 per cent chance of inheriting the gene and each grandchild a 25 per cent chance. From the study of many families it appeared that the gene could be carried by the male line with no effect on the men. It also appeared that a few women, such as one of my more distant family members, must be gene carriers because cancer appeared in their mother and one of their daughters. However,

---

[1] First-degree relatives are parents, siblings and children; second-degree are grandparents, grandchildren, uncles, aunts and half-siblings. First cousins are third degree.

these women do not develop cancer and are therefore examples of 'incomplete penetrance'.

Although it was generally recognised that a small proportion of both ovarian and breast cancers ran in families, it was still to be some years before any specific 'cancer gene' would be identified. There were, however, already a number of centres in the UK where there was active research in this area.

At that time the advice was that women at a 50 and 25 per cent risk of carrying the gene should be screened yearly with pelvic examination and abdominal or vaginal ultrasound, and that when they had finished having their families they may wish to consider having their ovaries removed.

In the letter from Cambridge I was also offered an appointment to speak to the director of the group, geneticist Bruce Ponder. This I did in September 1991. Dr Ponder was already an internationally recognised expert in the field, who had recently moved from London to establish the research group in Cambridge. In his late forties he combined his enthusiasm for research with a warm understanding of and wish to help affected families. Dr Ponder confirmed the conclusions that I had reached from the studies and my own research and explained further that my family history was clearly consistent with a dominantly inherited predisposition to ovarian cancer. As my nearest relative to be affected was my grandmother, my sisters and I had a 25 per cent chance of having inherited the gene, through my father.

Because I had almost reached 50 'without mishap', he said I had already gone some way to proving that I had not in fact inherited the gene. Research at that time suggested that my risk of being a cancer gene carrier would therefore have fallen from

25 per cent to about 18 per cent. As about 80 per cent of carriers eventually develop ovarian cancer, Dr Ponder calculated that my own risk of developing ovarian cancer before I was 70 was about 0.4 per cent per year or 1 in 12.

He went on to say that in most families with cases of ovarian cancer there are also some instances of breast cancer, more than would be expected by chance. So far this had not been the case in our family, so it could be that the predisposition in our family is only to cancer of the ovary. He warned me that we should nevertheless bear in mind this possible risk and consider appropriate regular breast cancer screening.

By then I had already decided to have my ovaries removed as a precautionary measure. He agreed that this was a very reasonable decision; even though my risk was not enormously high, it was clearly significant.

Following my appointment Dr Ponder sent me a comprehensive letter summarising our discussion and ending with 'If there are any questions that I can answer for you. . . I hope you will not hesitate to contact me.'

I appreciated this invitation and have repeatedly taken advantage of it over the years.

I told Felicity and Bunny of my discussions with Dr Ponder. As the chance of having children was now over for me, I would go ahead and have my ovaries removed. My sisters would have regular ultrasound screening. They might consider having their ovaries removed in the future. But not yet. Of their five children, the two youngest were then only three.

Meanwhile other members of the family were becoming concerned about their risks of cancer. My first cousin Molly is the daughter of one of my father's sisters, Helen. Helen, already in her eighties, had not developed cancer. She was therefore unlikely to be a cancer gene carrier, but it was still possible that she was one of the 20 per cent of carriers who do not themselves develop the cancer but can still transmit the cancer gene to their children. So Molly decided to have her ovaries removed. Her only other sister had already died from a malignant melanoma, unrelated to the family cancer gene.

The next person to be concerned was Molly's 24-year-old daughter. By now, we were all anxious to know whether there was likely to be a definitive test for the gene itself within the foreseeable future. It was clearly one thing to have major surgery if you knew you were carrying the cancer gene, quite another if you just might be, especially if in only a year or two gene testing became available and you were to discover the operation had been unnecessary.

By the end of 1991 the family was in a settled and happy phase. My father, now in his mid-seventies and retired from politics, was still involved with television and shipping companies and travelling the world. He and my stepmother, Cynthia, were regularly in London, and their Westminster flat continued to be a meeting place for their two combined families, as did the family home in Yorkshire.

Felicity was enjoying life with three young children, living in Kidlington, north of Oxford, in the large and beautiful Old Rectory. After spells on the *Financial Times* in Washington and *The Economist* in London, she had joined a literary agency in London. Recently she had left this to start her own agency in Oxford so that she could be more available to the children. Her husband, Alex, was working in Oxford and overseas as an agricultural economist.

Bunny with her two young daughters and husband, Rob, had just moved into a new house with a large garden, in the centre of Birmingham. Rob was the vicar in that parish and Bunny was helping him with parish duties. Bunny's Christian faith was central to her life and thinking. Soon after she left university, when she was working as a teacher in West Africa, she had sensed that she had a calling. She hoped that one day she would be a priest and had completed the training. As a deaconess, she had been the first woman teacher at Cuddesdon theological college and was now a deacon. Her attitude to the sexism she encountered was that example and steady persuasion, rather than confrontation, would win through. This was something that Felicity, active in the early women's lib movement, found hard to take and they had heated arguments about it.

Ronald and I were pleased with our recently enlarged cottage in the Golden Valley in Herefordshire. I spent a few days in London most weeks, at the Multiple Births Foundation, then in its most active and rewarding period. Otherwise I spent time writing at home or travelling and lecturing.

Ronald had finished his second book on how to resolve the Cold War, and was writing freelance as well as directing an educational charity on international security, Dunamis, at St James's Church, Piccadilly in London. He was often free to accompany me on overseas trips when we would try to add some extra days for a spell of holiday to the working programme. Luckily his appetite for art galleries and museums has always been greater than mine, so this could be largely satisfied while I was at the meetings.

Unusually that Christmas of 1991, we were scattered

between Birmingham, London, Yorkshire and South Africa but we were looking forward to a large family reunion in the New Year. Little did we realise that the shadow that had hovered over us for the last 15 years was about to become a reality.

Part Two
Close to Home

3

Coming Close to Home

IT WAS THE day before New Year's Eve, 1991. Ronald and I were alone at home; a lull between the festivities of a family Christmas in Yorkshire and the New Year on the Welsh border. The telephone rang. It was Bunny from a hospital bed in Birmingham. 'Lib, I've got cancer'. Her voice was soft but strong and calm.

She had been ill with what was thought to be bronchitis for the previous 10 days. We were concerned for her as she struggled to give her young children (aged six and three) the usual excitements of Christmas, as well as supporting Rob, who as vicar of a Birmingham inner city parish had his most demanding week of the year. They were always generous in opening their home to neighbours who might otherwise be alone at this time of the year. I had assumed that these pressures were contributing to her slower than expected recovery.

Now she told me the whole story. When antibiotics had failed to clear the bronchitis, she had been sent for a chest X-ray. This showed that she had fluid on her lungs and when this fluid was tested it contained cancer cells.

I was bewildered and shocked. Bunny was only 43. No one

in the family had had cancer so early in life. Despite intellectually accepting the risk we ran, I realised that I had never really expected it to happen to us. Furthermore, on the rare occasions that I did think about cancer, I had assumed that I, being the eldest, would get it first.

It turned out that Bunny was less shocked than we were. She wrote in her unpublished writings 'Lay Hold on Life':

> The news did not come as a great shock. I felt that I had already been prepared, partly through my own sense of disorder in my body – and partly, I am sure, because God prepared me.
>
> I had a dear lady in the bed next to me on Ward 20. She asked me what was wrong with me and when I told her she burst into tears. I was very touched by her response and it also made me realise just how serious it was.
>
> Rob came to see me that first evening – and he was just full of love – and also of thankfulness for all that we had shared in our lives. He seemed very strong and without fear.
>
> Right from the moment of discovery I had a sense that this had not happened by chance – but was all within the love of God and that His timing was perfect. Our sabbatical year was a lesson in God's provision. In so many ways He had supplied our needs – the house, the money, a new job. It was impossible to believe that somehow the illness was not also part of His plan.

Felicity was stupefied by Bunny's suggestion that somehow her illness was part of God's design. But unlike the arguments of the past, this time she bit her lip and said nothing.

From early in her illness Bunny had wanted to write of her experiences. She deeply believed that good would come out of it, that love would grow. She was keen that her thoughts should be shared with others and we, of course, encouraged her. She continued writing right into the last week of her life.

She describes her feelings in the early days after diagnosis:

One night – a few days after I had discovered about the cancer – I lay in bed feeling very weak and wondering if I could have the courage to journey forward. And I felt as if I heard a voice very close to me saying quite clearly 'All this is happening so that love may grow'. And already I know that love has grown – particularly amongst the family.

My father came to see me after I had been in hospital for three days. He looked so distressed and so old and, although it was awful to see him so upset, it made me realise how much he loved me and that was very precious.

It was clear that a cancer had spread to Bunny's lungs but at first the doctors were not sure where the cancer had started. Extensive tests and ultrasound scans were performed during the first few days. These showed that the ovary was the primary site. This was likely to be the same type of cancer that had killed our grandmother and aunt as well as a number of more distant relations. It was the first indication that my father must have inherited the family cancer gene.

Bunny continued:

The one bad moment was when a registrar surgeon informed me [on the Friday] that I would probably be having a hysterectomy on Monday. I had no warning that I might have surgery at all, so that was quite a sense of panic that the medical 'arm' might not know what the surgical 'arm' was planning. I insisted that I was allowed home for 24 hours to get life sorted out.

And so I came home, and Rob and I sorted out the girls' pants, vests and tights and tried to plough through some of the Christmas mess. But it was important to be home just for that night and to reassure the girls that I was all right.

On the Sunday morning Rob drove me back to hospital. Somehow the 'corner' that I had there has very precious memories for me – it became the place where I was surrounded by cards and flowers and where I felt utterly enfolded in the love and prayer of so many. I didn't want many visitors – but the sense of the unseen presence of so many dear friends was what I needed most.

The family came to see me – Libby was a wonderful comfort – and the girls came for the first time two days after my operation – Elizabeth keen to sort out all my cards and Catherine keen to find my food!

I wasn't afraid of the operation. I felt a great calm, which really carried me through that week. Looking back, the physical side was quite painful and difficult but somehow I was given great strength to deal with it.

Unusually Felicity and her family had not joined the Yorkshire family gathering for Christmas. They were in South Africa. Felicity's husband, Alex, had been brought up there, but had had to leave with his family when he was 13. Now things had changed and Mandela was free. Alex was taking his children for the first time to discover their roots. Bunny was anxious that this landmark holiday should not be interrupted. She asked us not to tell them of her illness; my father agreed with her. I had to accept the decision but found it difficult. Putting myself in Felicity's place, I felt I would have been very upset. I was wrong. They were grateful and more realistic than I. They knew that there was nothing they could have done in those early days. Their role in the months to come, helping with Lizzie and Catherine, would be much more important. Had Felicity been told she would almost certainly have taken the next plane to Birmingham.

It was agreed that I should send a letter to Felicity to await her return so that she would hear immediately but be able to digest the facts a little before she spoke to Bunny.

She returned to Oxford on the morning of 9 January 1992 with her three children, then aged nine, eight and four, all frazzled after a difficult and delayed journey. In fact, she had not had time to deal with the mail by the time I telephoned, so she hadn't read my letter. She drove straight to Dudley Road Hospital in Birmingham. By now Bunny was making a good recovery from the surgery.

Felicity remembers Bunny's urgent encouragement that she should have her ovaries removed. She had told her that 'with children you cannot take the risk'.

Lizzie and Catherine had missed out on their New Year visit to Yorkshire and now their seventh and fourth birthdays were due the following week. The grandparents invited them to celebrate these in Yorkshire together with their cousins, as well as Ronald and me, thus allowing Rob and Bunny to have time alone. Felicity, Alice and Max spent the whole of Thursday making an enormous *Treasure Island* birthday cake.

Although Bunny made an excellent recovery from her surgery she was under no illusion that she was cured of her cancer. She knew that if the cancer had spread to the lungs then the chance of a complete cure was very small, only about 5 per cent. She accepted this calmly and realistically but was determined from the start that she would give it her best try. If there was a 5 per cent chance of cure, why should she not be one of those lucky few? Anyway every year, every month, was worth living for, striving for, not least with such young children.

She coped very well with the six months of chemotherapy despite tiredness and nausea. Friends rallied round and helped with the children and Felicity or I often had them for weekends or during the holidays. Being similar ages, Felicity's three and Bunny's two were more brothers and sisters than cousins. And Lizzie and Catherine loved their older 'sister' Alice.

Meanwhile Felicity and I were anxious to get rid of our hazardous ovaries as soon as possible. We agreed that, for Bunny's sake, we shouldn't both be out of action at the same time. I had already been booked to have my hysterectomy and ovaries removed in the February and this went ahead uneventfully. Felicity's operation followed six weeks later. There was something quite satisfying to have the alternating patient/visitor role in our different hospitals and to compare experiences and the various hospital comforts or otherwise. Felicity and I visited Bunny and then each other. By the time that Felicity was in hospital Bunny had then recovered enough to visit her.

Felicity and I were both enormously relieved that our ovaries, when looked at under the microscope, were clear of any signs of cancer. We both admitted afterwards that we were convinced that we too had cancer as we had both had strange abdominal pains, presumably psychosomatic, in the weeks leading up to our operations.

As I was entirely healthy before my hysterectomy, I had assumed that I would recover quickly and be back to work without problems. I did make an entirely straightforward recovery and went back to work after six weeks, but was surprised at how tired I felt. It was at least a year before I regained my previous energy. I found this disconcerting and wished I had been forewarned. Too often doctors, particularly surgeons, are over-optimistic in their reply to the question 'when will I be back to normal?' If I had been told it would take 12 months I would have felt a sense of achievement had I managed by the eleventh. As it was, having been told three months, I felt a feeble failure for the following nine.

There was however one quite unexpected bonus to my hysterectomy. Although already 49, I realise now that I had never completely excluded the possibility of a 'miracle' baby. This was absurdly unrealistic but nevertheless I couldn't convince myself of it, especially as it was a recurring dream. To have removed all chance of ever becoming pregnant again was a surprising relief. At last I could really move on.

After the six months of chemotherapy Bunny appeared to return to full health for the next 18 months. She resumed a busy and full life as a mother and vicar's wife. She also, as a deacon, had her own church duties as well as some work as a chaplain in the hospital.

Bunny and I saw a lot of each other during this time. Not only did she bring the children over to Herefordshire quite often, but I also ran a monthly twins clinic in Birmingham, so I would always call in for tea afterwards and often spend the night with the family.

Although I knew that there was a high risk of Bunny's cancer recurring, she herself was so positive that I think we were all lulled into a sense of unjustified optimism. Perhaps that was good because there is no doubt that this was a very happy time for the whole family and any whiff of a cloud was high in the sky.

Throughout 1993 Bunny remained well. In August of that year it was my father's eightieth birthday party in Yorkshire. Bunny gave the speech, the grandchildren did a special cabaret, and we all danced until one o'clock in the morning with many old family friends.

The following month 30 of us joined Rob and Bunny to celebrate their tenth wedding anniversary with an Afro-Caribbean meal and a bouncy castle. Ronald gave a moving speech and we all felt it was a time of celebration and thanksgiving for her recovery.

But cancer had not left the family agenda. The year before, in 1992, Ronald had been referred to skin specialist because of a suspect mole on his right shin. The specialist immediately diagnosed a primary melanoma and called it 'alarming'. He said its swift excision was crucial and the operation was performed in a Plastic Surgery Unit outside Birmingham.

This time it was Bunny's turn to visit Ronald.

Initially I was, of course, shocked and also somehow confused. Another cancer in the family, unrelated to the hereditary ones, seemed unfair. However we were assured that Ronald's melanoma had been fully removed and that we could be very hopeful of a complete cure. By the time of Rob and Bunny's wedding anniversary, Ronald seemed to be fully recovered.

The following year, 1994, started less well. As Bunny wrote in her diary:

Sunday, 20 February 1994

It is now three weeks since I heard that my cancer has recurred and already I have started chemotherapy and am back in the system of hospital appointments and blood tests, and that strange nausea which is difficult to describe. I have wanted to write about this strange journey as honestly as I can. I think it will help me, and I hope and pray that it could help others too.

I knew that something was wrong. I had some strange stomach pain – and I am not a painy sort of person. I saw my GP who thought that it could be some infection but I think we both realised that it could also be a cancer pain. He gave me some antibiotics but the pain didn't go away and I knew, with that strange intuition that our bodies have, that it was definitely cancer.

On the Friday of that week I was due for my six-weekly hospital appointment with Dr Earle, my [oncology] consultant. I told her of my pain. It was then that she revealed that the 'tumour marker' – a particular blood test which shows the growth rate of cells – had been suspiciously high for some time [eight months]. I realised that the consultant I had seen before Christmas had tried to tell me this, but he had been too positive in his approach for me to take him seriously.

I found myself feeling quite angry with Dr Earle that she had not been more truthful about her suspicions. I asked why she had not told me; after all I had always said that I wanted her to be totally honest with me. She said that she had 'agonised' about whether to tell me and had then decided that, as I was so well, and as I did not ask, she would wait and see.

On reflection I am thankful for Dr Earle's decision. Last year was a wonderful year [and would have been] spoilt with the shadow of my illness. But now we talked about it. She was not able to find any obvious problem but we agreed that I would have the usual blood tests and then I would get in touch to hear the result.

The next few days was a strange time of waiting, a sort of limbo, knowing the truth of the situation in my own body but without clear medical confirmation. On the Saturday it was our PCC [parochial church council] away day. It was a very good day. . . most importantly there was a sense of love and care for each other. I was strangely aware that my illness was, in God's timing, somehow part of this process of learning to love one another more deeply and share our cares and concerns. Rob and I will certainly need this committed group to bear us along in our own vulnerability.

When I was ill, two years ago, the girls were cared for by many good friends. I have a strange knowledge that much of this was a re-run, of preparation. Now we have the assurance of that network of friendship and help which is close at hand.

I continued my limbo state until the following Friday when I went to see Dr Earle. She told me that the blood tests showed a high reading of 300 [the normal being under 50] and this confirmed her suspicion of cancer.

We then had an almost surreal conversation as I faced what this meant. I needed to understand as clearly as I could. She found it strangely difficult to tell me. I thought of all the many times she must have had to impart devastating news to patients or their relatives, perhaps it never gets easier for the doctor.

She told me that we were now talking of containing rather than curing the cancer, [that] it was possible to have chemotherapy because two years had passed since the outset of the last treatment [and] that those with ovarian cancer were usually relatively well until a few months or even weeks before their final illness. I asked her how I would die, and she said that people died of a blockage in the bowel caused by cancer growth. I asked the final question: how long did she think I had to live? 'I hope you will see the year through', was the reply [It was now late January].

It had been a difficult conversation for both of us but I felt good that I had asked all the hard questions, and that she had replied clearly.

When she left me in the little treatment room I swore like a trooper! I felt a gritted determination that I *would* do better than they said, much better than your average ovarian cancer patient. That's pride for you!

When I left the hospital there was a strange sense of relief. I now knew the worst, which really I had known for some weeks. But now it was clear, clinical and I understood the enemy much better. It was also something that could be shared.

I had always thought, since the first onset of cancer, that it was possible to recover with courage the first time round, [but] that I would find it impossibly difficult to face it a second time. Now I *was* facing it and I did not feel devastated in the way I had expected. I felt strangely prepared, even though in my own mind I had believed that after two years of being well I had quite recovered. I can only put this sense of preparedness to God's grace.

Rob was wonderful. For someone who can be such a fusser about little things, he is utterly solid when it is anything important. He was loving, accepting of God's strange ways, and we prayed together, offering it all back to the One who suffers with us.

I did not want any fuss. It was obviously important to tell family and friends, but I didn't want the showers of sympathy I had experienced when first ill: cards galore, flowers and a binge of caring. All that had been lovely at the time and part of the drama of me being in hospital. Now I wanted a quiet constraint, it felt a very different journey that we were travelling. And, of course, I didn't want the children to know. How, anyway, could they believe that Mummy might die in a year's time when she seemed so well?

So we tried to tell family and friends in a quiet way, asking for no cards, although I really appreciated letters. I did not want the girls to feel that anything was different. But children are strangely intuitive creatures. That first evening Catherine, aged six, said to me as I tucked her in bed 'Mummy, I will love you for evermore,' a phrase she had never used before.

It was hard telling friends. I wanted to tell them myself partly because I wanted them to hear, or see, that I was still alive and kicking, and partly because I thought Rob might get the information wrong! Several people burst into tears on me, and I felt a strange observer of their grief, feeling I should be able to comfort them. During these first weeks I felt that several people had tears in their eyes all the time that they were talking to me and I just hoped that this would not go on in a sort of chronic way through my illness.

Although I vividly remember Bunny's first illness, the diagnosis of cancer and the subsequent months, when it recurred much of this period is a blur. There are just islets of clarity. One was our Ash Wednesday service in Westminster Abbey. It must have been the children's half-term, just a few weeks after the realisation that Bunny did not have long to live.

She and I went to the early morning service. I did not pray for her recovery nor even much for her. My prayers were almost entirely selfish, or at least indirect, that I and the rest of her family and friends should know how best to support her, Rob and the children, to be given the strength to do this.

My family have been good. Libby my eldest sister is a wonderful support and it's a great comfort that she is a doctor. My only worry for Libby and for myself, is that she is so instinctively responsible and conscientious that she will feel a burden in getting her caring 'right'. When we shared a precious Ash Wednesday service she said afterwards that it was so important that we as a family live the illness in the right way. I so agree, but I feel I can trust that to God and I don't want her to worry about it.

I prayed, too hard it seems. One of Bunny's great strengths throughout her illness was to be able to become detached from it and to look not only at herself but at the needs of others. She was always very keen that cancer should not become her identity, that she shouldn't be 'the young mother with cancer' or the 'woman priest with cancer'. Unlike so many patients who become disempowered by their illness, Bunny somehow seemed to gain strength from it, psychologically if not physically. She was rarely demanding but knew what she wanted and what she believed to be right both for herself and for others. She remained quietly in charge until the end.

Of course her constant concern was for the children. And here she knew that Felicity's support would be vital. 'Felicity is just wholeheartedly generous,' she wrote. 'I know that she would help in any way she could. My children love her children and she will be able to help having the girls to stay, etc. So that is a great reassurance.'

Felicity, Bunny and I were worried about my father. He adored all three of us and Bunny was the youngest. He had been profoundly shocked by her first round of cancer; he would be even more upset now. I was worried too that he might, however illogically, feel responsible for, even guilty about, her cancer. It was almost certainly one of his genes that was responsible. In my work I am used to parents feeling responsible for the disability, the illness, or the death of their child, be it from an inherited disease, some damage in the womb or from some illness they have acquired in childhood. Rarely could any of these situations have been avoided, certainly not by any action on the part of the parents, and yet many parents carry an irrational guilt for ever.

Fortunately my father did not appear to suffer in this way. He was always a pragmatist, a realist. He was aware of the family genetics and where the gene came from. And as the years went by fate was to remind him of it only too often. But he rarely referred to it and I doubt that the fact that the gene came from his family rather than my mother's in any way increased his distress.

Of course Bunny knew that he would be shattered by her news. She writes:

I was worried about my father. He was abroad when I first heard the news so it seemed right to write to him, and give him time to digest it. But it was a difficult letter; I wrote with some trepidation. But when he rang me on return from his holiday he sounded strong, and later he wrote me a very special letter, which I treasure.

He said that I was born brave and that my faith had made me 'invincible'. That was such a strong word and made me quite determined to live up to it. He is a man who knows about bravery, and the times when courage fails. I remember him once saying that it was easier to be brave in your first battle than in your tenth. I hope I won't find that to be so in my illness.

Bunny had been working in the church for many years, first as a deaconess then, since her ordination in 1987, as a deacon. She was now waiting eagerly to join the first group of women in Britain to be ordained as an Anglican priest. Although a gentle and modest person she was, and was generally recognised to be, an excellent preacher. As our father said in his autobiography:

Bunny turned out to be a good, at times almost brilliant, preacher. As she has a low voice and speaks slowly she by nature avoids the two main hazards of women speakers, who tend to have high voices and speak too fast. She also speaks in parables and stories which hold your attention so much more easily than worthy exhortations.

As someone who often had to speak in public, I admired her quiet confidence and trust that she would find the right words. When we were both due to give tributes at our grandmother's funeral, I prepared mine well ahead, rehearsing it many times. Bunny was still composing her tribute in the car up to York and then gave an articulate and unfaltering performance. Now, perhaps for the first time, Bunny was to be anxious about a sermon.

The meeting with Dr Earle had been on a Friday, and on the Sunday I was due to preach at our main service. I wanted to do so, but wondered whether I would cope, so I rang two or three people asking them to pray for me. It's difficult to describe, if you have not experienced it, what it feels like to be surrounded in prayer but that is how I felt on that Sunday morning, and it was not difficult to preach.

During the service, as I was looking at the beautiful stained glass window of Christ above the altar, I remembered those words in the Gospel, 'Jesus set his face to Jerusalem'. It was the beginning of his journey to Jerusalem when all that lay ahead of him was suffering and death. I felt that in some sense He wanted me to 'set my face to Jerusalem', but this was not a morbid thought, rather a knowledge that the journey would be with him and after all, His journey had been a long one, full of encounters and diversions, and life. Cancer is such an invading illness that it is a wonderful comfort to know that this strange journey is in God's hands and that He has travelled a frightening journey as well.

Bunny had always had a large circle of friends, many with whom she kept in close touch; most of these friendships had been further strengthened by her first illness. Within her own family she tended to be the instigator of social activities. What with this band of friends as well as us family, I never doubted that she would have as many people there to help as she could cope with. Rob was a much more private person and, like many men, less prone to talking about his feelings. I worried that he might not have the same degree of outside support. Both his parents, who had been devoted and 'hands-on' grandparents, had died of cancer in the previous three years and his only brother lived far away.

But it was clear that he and Bunny gained strength from each other:

A week or so later Rob and I went out to a Chinese restaurant clutching a large bottle of wine. We needed time to talk together and we have often found that our best conversations have been when we go out to a meal. I can be quite honest with Rob. He loves truth and openness, which I find very liberating, so we talked together about our situation. We realised that Dr Earle had actually given me very little medical hope. It seemed I was expected to die within the year. We had two young children and Rob's job was an awkward one for a single parent. So we needed to face the future squarely. What would he do if I became ill and died? Should he leave his job as vicar of the parish, and if so how else could he earn some money? It was the job he had done all his adult life.

We ate our sweet and sour pork without solving any of the future. It seemed uncharted and impossible territory, but it was an extraordinary comfort just to be together and name the problems.

I reacted to the bad news in various ways. One of them was to be determined, very determined, to have lots of fun, a real desire to 'eat, drink and be merry', and to have a special time as a family together. The children and I were going to London for a few days for their school half-term and so we went on a shopping spree for clothes and bought two smart outfits. . . [When we got there] we explored the Natural History Museum with Libby, wandered around London Zoo, went to the British Museum, had some delicious meals and got to know the Underground better!

We had talked of going abroad for a holiday; now I was determined that we should do so. I have a step-brother, Patrick, and his wife, Ali, living in La Rochelle, so they were to be the beginning of a French holiday followed by Eurocamping and, if Rob could possibly face it, Euro Disney. So I put some energy into planning this as a sort of ordination celebration, to go for two weeks after I was ordained priest at the end of May.

So there was an instinct for life in all its fun and fullness, but also a deep anxiety about preparing to die. I am not a very practical person and certainly not at all systematic. If faced with the prospect of death I expect other people might worry about relationships, or work, or the process of dying – but I worried about untidy cupboards, a muddled desk and unfinished photo albums! I was also very concerned to get the house properly decorated – especially Catherine's bedroom. And these things really burden me – but perhaps it is easier to worry about untidy cupboards than something more profound.

I kept trying to imagine how Rob and the girls would manage without me. In my mind I wrote them a little recipe book with all the recipes that I knew – not a great repertoire, but at least it would be familiar. I tried to imagine how they would cope every day. But when I began to actually imagine how they would *feel* and the pain of the grief, it became quite unbearable and I went back to thinking about cupboards again.

Bunny was concerned too about the children's schooling, wanting to be involved in choosing their future secondary schools while she still had the energy. In other ways life went on apparently normally:

Quite often. . . I was an observer of myself – emotionally defended and constrained. I had had a long training from childhood in suppressing emotions; it was easier to be brave and positive than not to be so. The harder thing was to enter into the reality of the grief and pain.

I was not angry with God – or with anybody else – but I was grateful to other people who were angry on my behalf. Several friends told me how angry they felt – and they were clearly battling it out with the Almighty. Catherine's godmother came to visit us and sensed, as we prayed together, that the family was as safe as in a boat with a storm tossing around it. The storm represented the grief, anxieties and anger of other people that we were not to be overwhelmed by, but rather remained safe and together in the boat of God's love. I found this a helpful picture, a reminder that our life together as a family was all-important.

Looking back I realise that in those first few months I didn't hope and pray very assertively for healing. I believed that I would do better than medically expected but I had accepted the prognosis of death in a way that later I understood to be fatalistic and resigned. I think this was partly because I was struggling to understand God's ways, and wanting to be wishing to walk His way, whatever that meant. It was also because I did not want to deny the truth. I wanted to live it. And if the truth was that I only had a short time to live, then I wanted to plan to live well as well as to die well.

Within a few days of the recurrence being recognised Bunny started another course of chemotherapy. This was much less demanding than the first, a lower dose and less often. The pain settled and she felt fine. She wrote that:

this made the whole experience surreal. I could hardly believe there was anything wrong with me. When I looked in the mirror there I was – hale and hearty.

I learnt that friends and family tend to echo what you tell them. If I had said that I expected to be healed I'm sure they would have encouraged me. As I didn't they stood by me in what seemed to be an inevitable process. One or two people did challenge me. . . I was very often aware of the prayers of others. Sometimes I would sense a particular person praying for me – and that was quite wonderful and humbling too.

I have never been keen on large healing services unrelated to the ordinary life of the Church – or the razzmatazz that sometimes goes with them. I have also understood the local Church to be the body of Christ where all the gifts of His love and grace can be found so I had not looked for any other healing ministry than that of our own Church with its monthly healing service and faithful prayers. But three different people mentioned to me the name of John Petty, Provost of Coventry Cathedral, as someone with a particular ministry of prayer with cancer patients.

Accompanied by three friends, Bunny went to a service taken by

John Petty. She found it immensely moving and afterwards joined him for tea, where she had a conversation which she described as the 'turning point':

Having told him the story of my illness he said 'Bernadette, you are preparing to die and you mustn't. I have known other people with a similar prognosis who have been completely healed and you must believe that you can be as well. I don't believe that God would want a mother with young children to die.' I felt quite jilted and lovingly chastised. I also realised, almost immediately, that he was right. I had been preparing to die and after all I was still perfectly well.

Jesus was struggling with the thought of dying the night before He died, and I had been accepting it a year before when I was still reasonably well. I told John that I had been anxious to be prepared because of Rob and the children. But he assured me that I would be given enough time to prepare if and when that was needed.

I went away feeling very deeply stirred, not yet able to grasp the hope that I had been given. . . that I must want life for myself (not for the girls or Rob or the parish but for me). This was challenging and disturbing. Surely I *did* want life for myself. I had been fighting for it for the last two years, so I thought. . . That evening as I was washing up and pondering on the healing service, I had a very vivid picture of Abraham climbing with young Isaac up the mountainside. The old man was walking along with a dogged determination, obedient to the Lord ready to sacrifice the most precious thing he had, his only son.

When he came to the place of sacrifice I saw a lamb caught in the thicket and I heard a voice say, 'Jesus died so that you might have life.' And I realised, with wonderful clarity, that this was a message for me. God gave his very life away so that I might have new life. I did not need to die; I did not have to offer myself as any kind of sacrifice. This was mistaken obedience – a sort of false martyrdom. He wanted me to *live*!

From that day onwards I experienced a quite new sensation in my body, a sort of energy – an adrenalin – which I can only believe was healing. That Sunday the resurrection joy of Easter was very real to me.

The following days and weeks were a relishing of this new life. In the week after Easter we stayed at our little family cottage in Yorkshire and I felt well and essentially hopeful. The verse of a Wesleyan hymn came to me with great impact: 'Lay hold of our life and it shall be / Thy joy and crown eternally'.

The emphasis was on action – on *laying hold* of life. I was to put aside all that was passive or fatalistic and strive forward with a new assertiveness. And I found that I wanted this new life in quite a new way.

One day (when I was walking alone during our holiday on the [North Yorkshire] Moors) some words from Keats 'Ode to a Nightingale' came to me: 'for many a time I have been half in love with easeful Death'. The words shocked me because I realised that they referred to me and that somehow a part of myself had accepted the idea of death without a fight, even as a gentle exit from the struggle of life.

This was deeply disturbing as I had never believed it of myself. I thought generally I was positive and life affirming but somehow this negativity had crept in.

As soon as the words from Keats came to me, I thought of my

mother, and of the long and painful struggle she had had with death as a manic-depressive. Certainly she must often have been in love with easeful death. Somehow I had imbibed over the years some of my mother's longing to die. I had been very close to her as the youngest of her children. I was 12 when she became ill and before that she seemed to me everything that was good and life giving.

I realised that day that, just as my mother had been 'in love with easeful death', I must put any such thinking far, far away.

But it was not so easily done. Several weeks later I was to go on the ordination retreat for those of us women in the Dioceses of Birmingham who were to be ordained priest. The retreat was taken by Susan Cole-King, herself an Anglican priest. One of the first tasks she gave was on the importance of recognising our wounds, which we bring from the whole of our lives. We were encouraged to look at our own particular wounds which we brought to our ordination, and I found that grief and sadness for Mum were still heavy upon me, however far away I had thrown the temptation towards 'easeful death'.

One of the stories we were asked to reflect upon was that of the little girl who was presumed dead and whom Jesus raised to life. As I pondered on that little girl, Jairus's daughter, it struck me that she was 13 years old when Jesus raised her to life, just the age I had been when my mother became ill. I realised also that with Mum's illness a part of me had died, certainly my childhood had died and all the joy and freedom of that childhood.

I talked about this reflection with Susan Cole-King and she suggested that I should identify with the little girl and act out this story in the quiet of my own bedroom. So I took courage, and did just that. As I did so I found that it was quite difficult to be 'raised to life'. Something in me was still holding on to 'easeful death'. But then I did get up and felt wonderfully refreshed and imagined myself going down to the lakeside to play with my friends, full of life and health. I then imagined Jesus with my mother and I had an overwhelming sense that all was over and she is so well, and there is no more pain and unhappiness – no more need for us to grieve. I felt that she was reassuring me that the past is truly over and she is at one with her heavenly Father. All is well.

Since then, the grief that I had carried for so many years has gone and one day, after the retreat, I realised with a start that I had fallen in love with life and didn't want to let it go.

On 21 May 1994 Bunny was ordained as an Anglican priest, in Birmingham Cathedral. All the family came to support and celebrate with her, no one prouder than our father. The contrast between his two closest priestly relatives, his own father and his daughter, must have made him smile. My grandfather was notoriously fierce, arrogant and dogmatic, the complete opposite of Bunny. She was one of a group of women ranging in age from 26 to over 70, many of whom had waited decades for this moment. It was a moving and historic occasion. Never again would there be a group of such diverse ages, nor one who had waited so long to become priests. All had persisted, some vociferously, others with patient determination, all with tenacity and faith. After such a long wait some would only have a short working life ahead of them. None, as it turned out, a shorter one than Bunny.

4

The Slow Farewell: Bunny's Terminal Illness, Death and the Aftermath

FOR THE REST of 1994 Bunny was happy and apparently well. It is only now that I really appreciate her strength in coping so positively with the hopes, fears and uncertainties that must have been with her every day, however well she concealed them.

Soon after Christmas that year she mentioned on the telephone that she had some pain in her back that woke her at night. The GP had diagnosed an unusual virus infection. In February 1995 she wrote in her diary describing:

> strange tummy pains again and I knew the cancer [was] back again. The doctor came to see me and said he thought it would be good if we could go on a family holiday and I immediately grasped on to this. It seemed a wonderful idea to go on a special family holiday and so I put quite a bit of energy into organising a trip to Crete.

But the pain in the back continued and:

> gradually got worse until before Easter time I felt quite desperate. Finally it was discovered that I had cancer in my spine. In some

ways it was a relief to know exactly what had been happening. It seems that it's very unusual to have cancer in the bones with ovarian cancer but then I seemed to have been unusual in the different ways the illness has shown itself so it didn't surprise me.

During the early months of 1995 I kept in close touch with Bunny and her family, regularly visiting them in Birmingham. Although the girls continued to do well at school and outwardly appeared to be coping well, I now found my own relationship with them difficult. There was none of the enthusiastic welcome that I had always had in the past. Gone were the eager telling of their doings and joint story reading in my bed. Lizzie clearly didn't want much to do with me. I felt they often resented my presence. I could well understand. They wanted their mother not only to themselves but for her to do the things that sometimes I was now doing for them instead.

In the early summer, Rob and Bunny did take the children to Crete. Given how quickly Bunny's illness was progressing it was a bold, courageous move, but she was determined that the children should have happy times to look back on. Travelling had become hard but Bunny was clearly very pleased to have done it. It was a brief respite from what was about to come. From then on:

there followed a very difficult summer with one problem after another. I had radiotherapy for my back and also for my bladder, which had become completely blocked up. The great success was that the bladder tumour responded so well that [there] was no further need for a catheter.

By now the school summer holidays had begun and as usual Bunny and her family went up to the cottage on the Yorkshire moors. Here she developed an obstruction of her bowel and was admitted to Scarborough Hospital, critically ill. I went straight up to join her there. It was apparent that she needed an urgent operation but also that she might not survive it. She was fully aware of this and prepared herself calmly. She decided to talk to each of the girls on their own and also dictated a message to them on her little hand Dictaphone.

I marvelled at how, with the same confidence as she gave her sermons, but now in pain and heavily drugged with painkillers, she dictated fluently the most beautiful and reassuring message to each child. Messages that were appropriate to their age and personality, yet ones they could continue to treasure. She looked forward with them to the way they would enjoy and use their own individual gifts and talents. Copies of the tapes were originally kept by Rob for the girls, and then given to them.

> When I was in the [Scarborough] hospital those words from years ago came back to me that 'this is all happening so that love may grow'. It was so much the right place to be for the family. I had a very special time with my father and with the rest of the family as well. It was a great blessing to be surrounded by the homeliness of Yorkshire love and voice which reminded me so strongly of my childhood. There was comfort too in Libby and Felicity sleeping by my bedside [in the hospital] and us talking together in the night like when we were children.

Patients when very ill vary so much in their needs. Some like to have times of peace and solitude. Despite her serenity and apparent lack of fear, Bunny did not like to be alone. We and other friends were of course happy to be with her and she was rarely without one of us by her side. Her niece Alice, aged 13, felt deeply for Bunny. She was a sensitive child, mature for her age, and we were slow to appreciate that she wanted and deserved to be part of the adult support team. It was comforting for them both when she was allowed to join the rota and spend time with Bunny.

For me this was a strange and precious time. Not only was I with Bunny, but I was also back in the hospital where I had spent my first rewarding and sometimes heart-rending year as a doctor. Vivid memories of my first patients flooded back, of my bedside vigil by one little five-year-old dying of leukaemia and of the old man who gave me 12 pots of honey to thank me for my help with his 'waterworks'. But mainly I was just so grateful to be in a hospital with warm and understanding staff who were happy to have me there all day and night. I even accompanied Bunny into the operating theatre in the early hours of the morning and waited in the anaesthetic room for her return. I felt as young and inexperienced as I had nearly 30 years earlier.

Yet again Bunny recovered better than expected but it was clear that she would not regain her strength. Pain control had now become the main aim. On the whole this was successful. Understandably, she and Rob wanted to get back to Birmingham, so that the girls could get on with their normal pattern of life and return to school at the beginning of term. So, three weeks after her operation, Bunny came down by ambulance to St Mary's Hospice in Birmingham. Apart from going home for her birthday, 26 September, and for the final weekend, she remained there, in the excellent care of all the staff, until she died.

During the last weeks she had one by one seen and said goodbye to her closest friends, to her brothers-in-law, Ronald and Alex, and to our father and stepmother. Each knew that this was a final farewell. Bunny gently and generously said her goodbyes without fear or embarrassment.

Wednesday 11 October 1995 Bunny wrote:

Today has been a very important day for me. It's been a day when I've realised just how ill I am but I've finally accepted it. In several ways I was jolted yesterday into recognition of the truth. The first thing was that my dear friend Hilary told me that she felt that she had been urged to pray in a different way for me. To pray that I'd be prepared for everything that God wanted to give to me now. To be prepared to die. The second was a lovely honest conversation with Libby who helped me to see how much I had been fighting the truth of the situation. The third thing was that last night I suddenly had a horrid attack of breathlessness. I've never experienced anything quite like it before but it really frightened me and I've since been told that this could be quite a dangerous sign of something that could be fatal another time.

I can only say that between last night and this morning a truly wonderful change has happened in me. I no longer feel the frustrated fight, the realisation that I'm not getting better and a longing to do so. I no longer feel that I've got to improve my walking and all the other things which seem to be getting worse at the moment. I feel a real peace, a sense of handing over into God's hands and that it's now possible to do that.

With that has gone a determination to tell the children as

much as I can and so today I saw each of them separately and said that as far as we understood I didn't have very long to live. I wanted them to realise that I am not improving. I didn't want to be living a lie in front of them. They were both wonderful in their own way and took it bravely. Now tonight Libby tells me that if I want to go home there is some sense of urgency because in fact the attack I had last night seems to have been particularly worrying and therefore it's important if I'm going home that I go home soon. So maybe it will be on Friday rather than Monday. I realise that my desire to be at home is to be with Rob and the children just for one short spell of time.

Through all the years of Bunny's illness, Rob had shown the most remarkable fortitude and resilience. Once when I said this to him, he replied that his experience at work, as a priest, had prepared him. I found that my own extensive experience of dying, death and bereavement as a doctor seemed to be of little help to me with my own sister. Rob rarely spoke of his own stresses or worries, although they must have been enormous. Towards the end my heart went out to him because he just couldn't be in two places at once and he must have longed to be in them both. He and Bunny must have yearned for more time together but they both felt the children must be the priority. No one could replace a parent at this critical time and sadly I could be no help except as a late-evening babysitter. The girls didn't want me around.

Luckily Felicity and I wanted to be with Bunny as much as we could. I knew how important it is for the dying person to be at peace with their carers. I know too that family are not necessarily who they want. Too often I have seen distressing tensions at the bedside of a dying person. Bunny and I had discussed this many months before and agreed that she should just guide us when the time came. Felicity and I were of course so happy that she wanted us there. But that may not always have been easy for Rob. We are very close as sisters and both Felicity and I can be organising and bossy. I realise there were times when we were tempted to take, or took, more control than we should have done.

Sometimes decisions were difficult. I knew that Bunny desperately wanted to go home for what turned out to be the last weekend of her life. She wanted to give the children the chance to relax with her and to talk if they wanted to. Lizzie in particular did not like visiting the hospice. Very understandably: it was where people were dying and an unwelcome reminder of how really ill her mother was. There were, anyway, much more interesting things for a 10-year-old to be doing.

We all knew it was a risk for Bunny to go home. Yet if she died there, there should be no regrets. For Rob it was particularly difficult. Although he had realised the importance of her coming home before she died, he was thrown by the putting forward of the date. He had heavy parish duties that weekend including a confirmation and he felt a responsibility towards the candidates he had been preparing. I could understand this but felt Bunny should make the decision and I wanted to support her in whatever that was. So preparations were made. Nurses were arranged, the air bed installed and some cushions were added rather precariously to the bed so that there was room for Rob as well.

On Friday 13 October Bunny went home for 48 hours. She had lovely talks with Lizzie and Catherine. When she returned on the Sunday evening she was content. She said that all she needed to do was now done and she hoped that she would die very soon.

On 16 October 1995 she wrote for the last time in her diary:

Today is Felicity's 50th birthday and she is with me as we write these final words. It is clear now that I have not got long to live and I have no fear of dying. In fact now that the time has come, I feel an impatience. I have fought the good fight as best as I have known how. So I 'lay hold on life and it shall be Thy joy and crown eternally'

'All things work for good for those who love God.'

Two days later she was ready to die, wanted to die, but somehow felt she was holding herself back. She knew that we were all as prepared as we could be, largely thanks to her gentle guidance. Prolonging her life now would not help her or indeed any of us. The emotional and physical strain would inevitably take a toll, particularly on Rob who was striving to keep some sort of normality in the children's lives. But how could Bunny help herself to take her leave?

We spoke openly to each other. I said I did not know the answer but wondered if she shouldn't just rest, cease planning (she had only just stopped ordering new nightdresses from Nightingales), stop giving attention to other people, stop making efforts of any sort. Was there anything more she wanted to say to Rob, to me, to Felicity or to anyone else? No. Then I suggested that she should now rest. One of us would be with her at all times but would ask no questions, nor try to engage her in conversation. She would just know that we were there and loving her all the time.

Most nights in this last week, Bunny slept well, only waking once or twice for brief words. But the final night was different. She was restless, muttering that she'd forgotten to pack her bag. In the morning she was again peaceful. Felicity meanwhile was driving from Oxford and later wrote:

I was doing my regular morning M40 run from Oxford to Birmingham diverting myself with the radio. Richard Hoggart was on *Desert Island Discs* and I remember he chose the great 'Prisoners' Chorus' from *Fidelio*, when the prisoners emerge from their dungeon into the light. I was driving along belting out 'O welche lust' with tears streaming down my face. And I remember thinking 'This is when Bunny is dying.' It was when she was being released into the light – which is funny when you think what an un-religious person I am. When I got to the hospital half an hour later I was surprised – almost put out – to find her still alive, though totally unconscious. And I remember all that day as I fussed around in her room I was talking to her in my head, but I was not talking to the figure on the bed any more.

In the afternoon Rob went to pick up the children from school but soon after he left Bunny's breathing became more erratic and then, with Felicity and me on either side of her, she suddenly and clearly left us. She died entirely peacefully.

Felicity and I hugged each other, wept, but were so relieved for Bunny. No one could have fought the good fight more courageously while still treasuring life and finally leaving it with a grateful faith in a new one. We were so thankful to share this last experience – it was unusual for us both to be by her bedside together – either of us would have been sad to have missed such a precious moment. Our only concern was that Rob should have been deprived of it.

In the long hours by her bedside, we had had plenty of time to help make plans for the immediate period after Bunny's death, many of them with Bunny's help. We had made lists of who should telephone who; what help, if any, we could give to Rob and the children; who should write the obituaries. Indeed these had already been written and were to be prominent in all the main newspapers. One newspaper said:

> At times she had grown impatient with the long and often bitter debate over women's ordination in the Church of England but she seldom gave way to righteous anger and instead substituted for it her own sense of wry amusement. When the moment of decision finally came she had absolutely no doubt about her desire for ordination, even though she was already gravely ill.
>
> *The Times* 25 October 1995

Another wrote:

> She was not a rabid campaigner but she spent her life gently and firmly breaking down the barriers against women's leadership in the Anglican church. She disarmed the opposition by her warmth, her gift of listening, her clear but untrumpeted abilities and the twinkle in her eyes. . . Her cancer. . . she faced and fought it with all the faith and joy that was in her. She claimed that 'you become more vibrantly alive when you face up to death.' When a friend referred to someone else as dying of cancer Bernadette retorted, 'She's not dying. Until we're dead, we're living.'
>
> *Guardian* 1 November 1995

Felicity and I had been in Birmingham almost continuously for the final two weeks and it was time for us to go home and to leave Rob and the children to grieve in peace. We knew that they would be well supported by many friends and neighbours in the parish.

Rob would make all the arrangements for the funeral and burial. Felicity and I, with help from our father and three of Bunny's friends, were to take responsibility for a thanksgiving service in Yorkshire a few weeks later.

The day after Bunny died, I was due to speak at a large meeting on Multiple Pregnancy at the Royal College of Physicians in London. I had participated in an earlier workshop, the proceedings of which were being published as a book. This conference was to present our findings. I had expected to have to cancel my presentation but now, with Bunny's death, there was no reason for me to do so. It was on bereavement following the death of a newborn twin.

I started by apologising for not being able to join them for the whole two-day meeting and told them why. I then pointed out how positive my experience had been in comparison to the parents I was to speak of. I had been able to say a loving farewell, knowing that all we wanted to say to each other had been said and knowing that I would always have happy memories to treasure for the rest of my life. In contrast these parents would have lost someone to whom they had had no chance to give their care and love, no time to create memories to treasure and no time to say goodbye.

Bunny's funeral service was held on All Saints' Day in Birmingham in their own parish church, St Luke's. The church was packed full of relatives, friends and parishioners. Seventeen women priests filled the choir stalls. After the service, in the autumn sunlight, we all drove over to the city graveyard on a hill. Led by a wonderful Afro-Caribbean choir, we sang hymns, sad and joyful, throughout the half-hour it took for the grave to be filled by the male relatives and friends. We sang and wept and hugged each other. The girls were surrounded by their young cousins and school friends. I prayed that this support would sustain them, especially if they found it difficult to accept ours.

Some months later a stone decorated with a Celtic cross was placed on the grave. Rob and the children deliberated over the inscription. Finally biblical texts were discarded following her children's suggestion that the most appropriate words should be those of Bunny herself: 'That Love May Grow'.

Meanwhile Felicity, unable to sleep, had gone to her GP for sleeping pills to help get through the funeral the following week. As she was there she asked him to look at a mole on her leg as she felt there was something odd about it. He agreed and wanted to remove it immediately.

She insisted on postponing the operation until the day after Bunny's funeral. Like Ronald's it proved to be a malignant melanoma. Although the specialist thought he had removed the entire cancer he was concerned that there were signs that it had spread to the lymph gland in her groin. Major surgery was indicated to avoid further and life-threatening spread of the cancer. She had this a few days later and was home in time for Christmas. She wrote:

> I remember keeping it all very quiet. I felt very embarrassed to have come up with this complication when everyone was mourning Bunny. So I told very few people and slunk into

hospital in mid-December – a time when I hoped nobody would notice. I didn't tell Papa till some time after and I don't think he ever really knew what had happened. It was so very confusing. I remember lying in the ward when the carol singers came through and crying my heart out. I didn't know what I was crying for: Bunny, myself, the fear that I might not live to look after the children. . .

During this time, I don't think I was myself conscious of grief, just a sense of huge relief that Bunny had been spared any more suffering and that the end had come so peacefully. Others shared their grief and their love for Bunny with us. As one friend wrote from Africa:

> I'm grieving for that rare inestimable quality of friendship that runs very deep, risks revealing, trusts boldly, but is also full of fun and laughter. Bun's friendship was a kind of healing for me, and a challenge to risk openness with others, realising how much I needed it from them.

Once the thanksgiving service in Yorkshire was over, we returned home to pick up lives that had been in limbo for many months. Meanwhile Rob, Lizzie and Catherine started their new life, one with many changes. We could only admire the strength with which they went forward. They moved house. Rob had always had a very demanding job and, apart from the ever-popular 'rough and tumble' episode before bedtime, had left most of the childcare to Bunny. Clearly childcare could not now be combined with the life of a busy vicar, particularly as so many parish activities are in the evenings or during weekends.

A big decision had to be made. Rob was clear that the right one was for him to give up this job, to move house and find lighter priestly work so as to be able to look after the children and the house. The alternative of having a housekeeper or a nanny was not one he wished to consider.

He was blessed with an unusually responsible and efficient helper in 10-year-old Lizzie. The only problem was that her domestic standards were so high and her views so strong that I would have found her a daunting accomplice. I sometimes worried to see the responsibilities she took upon herself. Both children have always had enormous energy and determination. Any emotional response to their mother's death was never shown by the apathy and loss of focus so common in depressed or grieving children. Rather, their determination seemed to increase, sometimes to an obstinate degree.

It must have been an agonising time for the girls. It was painful for me too. I had always been very close to them both, particularly Lizzie. From the age of two she had stayed with us on her own, sometimes bringing friends with her. I never expected or wanted a parental role in their lives, even when it looked as though Bunny might die when they were very young. But I had always cherished our close friendship. Now there was the added wish to do all and anything I could for Bunny's sake.

But there seemed little I *could* do. They didn't want me close. I don't think it was as difficult for Felicity. Inevitably her one-to-one relationship with the girls was less close than mine. She had rarely been alone with them as her own children were always around. Now her children could act as a buffer to any awkwardness between aunt and nieces. I had no one to soothe the tension of our relationship, just a husband who found it very difficult to understand these distant, often abrupt, children. Greetings, 'sorry' and 'thank you' were lost from their vocabulary. I was torn between wanting to avoid further alienation by not insisting on these social niceties and a husband who felt that discipline was called for. My own emotions were raw and I found it impossible to be objective. All my professional experience of helping parents to understand and cope with difficult behaviour in bereaved children was useless.

I couldn't even hug them. The children had been used to lots of cuddles and hugs. Bunny was a wonderfully affectionate and demonstrative mother. As little children they readily responded to the hugs and kisses of friends and relations. This was no longer so. Of course they were older but the change was abrupt and extreme. More than a peck from me would have been unwelcome. I could have accepted this, even if with sadness and perhaps jealousy, had I felt that the cuddles were coming from other adults. But it seemed that none of Bunny's women friends were able to get physically close. Nor did the girls have any grandparents nearby. The thought of these bereaved children never being lovingly embraced by a woman was agony. I knew as the Irish poet, John O'Donohue so beautifully puts it:

Touch and the world of touch brings us out of the anonymity of distance into the intimacy of belonging. . . It is recognised that every child needs to be touched. Touch communicates belonging, tenderness and warmth which fosters self-confidence, self-worth and poise in the child.[2]

[2] O'Donohue, John, *Anam Cara*, Bantam Books, London, 1999

I could only hang in there and hope that the barriers would gradually come down.

It is hard to imagine this period now. Both the girls have become generous huggers and any inhibitions in our relationship, either emotional or physical, disappeared several years ago. We have spent lots of time together at family gatherings and also on our own. We often regret that we don't have more time together. For an eighteenth birthday present Catherine and I spent three happy days in Barcelona. Lizzie has several times come to us as a helper for weekend gatherings.

With Lizzie, the breakthrough came when she was 14, four years after Bunny's death. I offered her a week's holiday in France. Ponies and a large swimming pool were the main carrots. She and I joined our close friends the Pietronis' annual house party in the Dordogne. Sixteen of us ranged in age from teenagers to those in their seventies and included several psychotherapists. Lizzie was the youngest and everyone loved her and made a fuss of her. The week was action packed and full of laughter and hugs. She adored it, begged to stay on a second week on her own, which she did. Just before I left, she and I went for a walk. We lay in a field and talked of the difficulties of the past few years. I still treasure that moment. With Catherine the breakthrough was more gradual but no less complete.

Over the years we have all three freely acknowledged our past difficulties but never discussed them in any depth. Last autumn I asked Lizzie if she would be prepared to do so now, not least to see what lessons could be learnt for helping children in the future.

Lizzie readily agreed. I emailed ahead to give her some idea of what I hoped we could talk about, then went down to Brighton where she is in her last year as a photography student. Over a delicious and prolonged Thai supper, we talked and talked.

I was surprised how little she remembered of her mother's illness. After the initial illness, she said she did not think of her mother as any different to anyone else's or not until the last few months of her life. She said things like: 'I never thought about it', 'it's a blank', 'awful', 'I was old enough to remember these things I've just blanked it out.'

Lizzie worries now that she had not given as much attention to Bunny as she should during the final months. At the time she just wanted to do something else, to be with her friends, but she now feels that subconsciously it may have been because she couldn't face the fact that her mother would soon die.

When I broached the question of her emotional inaccessibility and resistance to physical contact, she replied: 'Of course that's all I wanted really. In my mind I was annoyed with people for not trying to get closer. . . but how was anyone to know? It was a constant battle because I knew the way I was putting myself forward was stopping anyone having contact but I was also desperate for it. . . but couldn't work out how to show it and let my guard down. I knew I was making it difficult for everyone.'

Over 10 years later, she looks back remarkably philosophically, recognising not only the times of real pain but the positive things that have come out of the experience: an independence, deeper relationships, an increased understanding of other people and an acceptance and respect for their wide range of views and opinions. Because, as she said to me, 'everyone is so different. . . to be able to understand each other and ourselves is impossible and something we can only aim at.'

She doubts whether we could ever have got it right, but it would have been a huge comfort in those dark times to have known that one day we could have such a relaxed and happy evening together.

Catherine is currently spending her gap year in Chile teaching in a primary school in Chol Chol, nine hours' bus ride south of Santiago. I have not therefore been able to have the same focused conversation that I did with Lizzie but I sent her a draft of this chapter and asked her if she would like to add anything. This was her response:

In the first weeks after Mum's death I remember feeling very numb inside but not conscious of pain. It is hard for a seven-year-old to understand death. In the last stages of her illness Mum was either in bed or in the hospice; I saw less and less of her. When she died I didn't see her at all; it was not such a big shock because the change was gradual. I remember feeling guilty because I did not feel as sad as I was expected to feel. I also remember her featuring in my dreams.

One day, not long after the event, something particularly upset me; I lay on my bedroom floor and thumped it hard with my fists shouting 'I want to die! I want to die!' Dad found me and gathered me up in a bundle of tears, which is probably what I most wanted, even if I didn't realise it. Looking back I connect the wish to die with a wish to be with Mum and with my annoyance that I couldn't call her to me as I always had done. She had told me that I would see her in heaven just as she was going to see her mother.

As the months went on I became angry, I felt that I had not been made sufficiently aware of what was happening as Mum was dying; until the end I still believed she would get better. Even when she told me she was going to die very soon I'm not sure it really hit me. Looking back now I realise that the adults around me probably told me as much as they thought I could take.

I also regret not having seen Mum in the week before she died. It might have seemed natural not to bring such a young child to a deathbed, but it meant that the reality of what was happening didn't really dawn on me.

I do not recognise myself in your description of the difficult children who, 'didn't want me close'. I am not aware of having purposely or even consciously shunned attention, but I do not doubt that that is how it may have seemed. I know that I became a lot shyer after Mum died and with that came a feeling of clumsiness, awkwardness and not fitting in. I think I tried to grow up too fast. I was never intentionally rude to you as far as I can remember; I am sorry if I came across that way. For a long time I felt that you wanted me to be someone different and that made it difficult for me to be open with you.

I admired her insight and was grateful for her honesty. But of course I was saddened by our mutual misunderstanding. I certainly never wanted Catherine to be someone different. I loved her generous nature and admired her determination, but I did wish she could still show the warmth, enthusiasm and appreciation to others that she always had as a little child. I knew it was there but concealed by the shyness and awkwardness that she herself describes. In my misguided and, no doubt, overbearing efforts to encourage, I probably made it even harder for her. And at the same time I became increasingly less accessible to her.

Bunny's wish for those final two days at home was primarily so that, in a familiar environment, she could have peaceful time alone with each child and allow them to talk as freely as they felt able about their worries and fears. The question of how much and at what stage a young child should be made aware of the gravity of their mother's illness, and of how involved they should be in the terminal phase is always a difficult one. Not only may the adults in the family have different views on this, but the personality as well as the age of the child will influence decisions. Further dilemmas arise when the needs of the two children appear to differ. One may find comfort in being with their mother as much as possible while the other may be overwhelmed, even if unconsciously, by anticipatory grief and prefer the distraction of their own friends.

For how long should parents pretend that life will one day return to the same happy one that the children have always known? At what point should the true situation be shared with them? The balance between burdening young children for an unnecessarily prolonged period and allowing them sufficient time to understand and at least begin to prepare for their mother's death is not easy. Not least they will need time to raise all their questions and fears about how life will be without their mother and receive reassurance about how they will cope with the day-to-day practicalities of life.

If given the chance children can often take the lead themselves in saying or at least showing what they want. But many will not do so to their parents for fear of adding further to the family stress and sadness. A child may sometimes be happier to talk to a sensitive teacher or family friend who can then relay their wishes and, where appropriate, answer their questions.

As a paediatrician I have sometimes tried to help parents as they struggle to make these various decisions and to support their children through an experience that cannot fail to be agonising. It is so much easier to do this when one is not emotionally involved oneself.

Nine years after Bunny's death, the family again moved house to join Rob's second wife, Helen. This inevitably meant a big turn out and the further discarding of some of Bunny's clothes and possessions. Catherine, now 17, expressed her feelings of loss in this poem to her mother.

'Moving On'
They are coming on Wednesday.
They are coming on Wednesday to pack up.
They will take the old red sofa I hid behind
(whilst you played seeker).
It will go off to the dump.

They will take the plastic tablecloth and the table
Where you served my favourite, lasagna.
I do not like it anymore.

We have been through your clothes.
So many long dresses, African beads, Indian silks.
Pinks, reds, blues, outdated but still beautiful.
The ball gown that you wore for Grandpa's birthday
And the bright green jumper with the ducks on.
I remembered them.
Like picking up a once loved book;
Inside the pages were blank.

Singing the Life

Your perfume, your touch, has left them
They could not hold you back and neither could I.
They are musty and moulding, starched and folded in cruel lines
We must get rid of some,
We cannot take them all with us.
There are too many memories, too many lives,
How will the broken pieces make a whole?
In this new place.

We brought you to this house;
You smile at me from every wall,
There is your wedding dress in the wardrobe,
Your old records (no one listens to any more).
There will be new photos where we are going,
But not many.
No one remembers to take them anymore.

I have painted the bedroom 'aqua'
Even the ceiling
Sunshine ripples through the window
And splashes across my private lake.
On Thursday I will move in;
I will be in there sometime.

They are coming on Wednesday
Piece by piece they will pack our lives away.
Many things are going to the jumble sale
The stories you read to me and the roller skates for my birthday.
Many things of yours
Going where they mean little, cost less.

The Slow Farewell

And will you be boxed up with the rest?
Will you come with us a second time,
Or must I say goodbye again?

5

More Cancers and BRCA1

IN JUNE 1992, three years before Bunny died, I had an update on the current situation on 'predictive genetic testing' for family cancer from Maggie Ponder, the research assistant in Cambridge. She wrote about a pilot study that was planned on a few selected families known to be available for testing:

> The problems of pre-symptomatic genetic testing are quite comple . . . first you have to make sure that the test will definitely work and to begin with that will vary from family to family. Then you have to embark on explaining the test to the whole family, outlining the possible results and their implications. Having done that, those who wish to be tested will be invited to discuss it further before they finally decide, and they will need careful counselling at the time they get the results. . . The problem with ovarian cancer is that although those who get a negative test will be much comforted, those who test positive still have tricky choices to make about screening, [preventive] surgery, having children, etc.

A month later Bruce Ponder talked to me more fully on the

scientific background and specifically about the prospects for genetic diagnosis in our family. This took some digesting. The evidence suggested that about 90 per cent of breast/ovarian cancer families are due to damage to the gene on chromosome 17q. He explained that it must first be seen whether or not the ovarian cancer in our particular family is due to such damage. Once the site of damage is defined this information can then be used for testing other family members to see if they too carry the diseased chromosome.

He went on to say that our family was a little unusual in that, at least so far, it has, apparently 'site-specific ovarian cancer': the cancers had been limited to the ovary rather than also affecting the breast. This made it harder, in the state of knowledge at that time, to estimate the probability of the 17q gene being the one that was affecting our family, although it remained likely that it was.

Dr Ponder explained:

In this situation, one looks for confirmation of the suspected linkage from the inheritance of chromosome 17 markers with the family. The problem is that we have only samples from two affected individuals. . . They are quite distantly related [my sister and my father's first cousin] so in genetic terms this would be quite powerful, but only if our markers will define a haplotype[3] which is sufficiently uncommon that we can be confident that if they share it, it is actually because they have the same chromosome, rather than simply the same marker

---

[3] A haplotype is what makes up, genetically, each individual chromosome. It is used to ascertain whether or not a disease has genetic origins.

alleles[4] coming on to the family by coincidence from elsewhere in each case. . . in principle this may be possible, but we will need to have blood samples from the close relatives. . .

If the markers turn out well, I estimate that we might be able to provide genetic diagnosis with an accuracy of better than 90 per cent. . . At that point, of course, we have to confront all of the ethical issues and decisions. . . about who really wants to be tested, and how to handle the information. The general feeling in the genetics community is that a small well-defined pilot study should be done to find out more about these issues in practice, and we are planning this at the moment.

However, it was not until early 1999 that a mutation in the gene, by now named BRCA1, was identified in our family. Much was to happen before then.

A few years had passed since that conversation with Dr Ponder. It was now just over a year since Bunny had died. It had been a sad and difficult time but we were now all back to a regular pattern of life. Rob, Lizzie and Catherine had moved into their new home in Moseley in Birmingham and the girls were settling into their new school. Felicity had had no further trouble following the removal of the melanoma on her leg and Ronald was just approaching the fifth anniversary of the removal of his. Despite the oncologist's warning that melanomas, more than any other cancers, were notoriously capricious, indefinitely

---

[4] An allele is one of a series of DNA codes that occupy a specific position on a chromosome and are therefore useful to determine whether or not a disease is shared by members of the same family.

unpredictable, we had begun to relax. We were all beginning to feel we were in smoother waters.

But one morning in January 1998, Ronald said he could feel a lump in his groin. Within a few days an examination showed that his malignant melanoma had spread to at least that one lymph gland.

We were told that there was no knowing how far Ronald's cancer may have spread, that the outlook was worrying and that the only hope lay in major surgery – an inguinal and iliac lymph node resection, which means clearing lymph nodes in the groin and right up into the abdomen. Even then the chance of five-year survival would be only about 50 per cent. If, during the operation, it was found that the cancer had spread to other glands, beyond the groin, then the outlook would be much darker still.

We had also been told that this operation was not one routinely performed in our local Hereford hospital. What should we do? There should be no delay. It was to our good friend Patrick Pietroni we turned for advice.

It was not long since we had first met Patrick and Marilyn Pietroni. At the time Patrick was a GP in London and had recently established the Marylebone Health Centre, a pioneer project in which a range of complementary therapies and counselling was integrated into an NHS general practice. Marilyn had been a social worker and was working at the Tavistock Clinic as a psychotherapist.

The four of us met when spending the weekend together with Jenifer Wates, the recently widowed wife of Neil Wates. We were gathered to discuss how a trust created in Neil's memory might best be used to help future cancer sufferers.

We were all grieving, shocked and vulnerable. Marilyn and I were, after prolonged struggles, each trying to come to terms with never now having our own children. Patrick and I had both come off the orthodox medical career ladder and started our own projects, his much more ambitious than mine, but we shared many of the same emotions of doubt, excitement, and uncertain funding. For many years, as well as running Dunamis, Ronald had been involved as Chairman of the Champernowne Trust for psychotherapy and the arts. We were amazed by the range of our shared interests and experiences, and the synchronous timing of them.

By the end of the weekend a firm friendship had developed. The Pietronis have remained among our very closest friends and there is no couple to whom we have turned for more help, advice and support and continue to do so throughout this present long, as yet unfinished, saga.

Now Patrick advised Ronald to see an oncology surgeon in Harley Street. He was admitted to a London teaching hospital for surgery the following week.

To our intense relief the pathology reports showed that there was no sign that the cancer had spread to the internal lymph glands. Gradually Ronald recovered from the operation but because of an MRSA infection his stay in hospital was prolonged to nearly four weeks, with several more weeks in bed at home.

Ronald and I had both had previous experiences of hospital care in which there was a real team spirit among the ward staff, teams who had worked consistently together and who encouraged each other in the highest standards of care, hygiene and continuity. Now Ronald witnessed an ever-changing relay of agency and other nurses who sometimes had to ask him about his condition and treatment. This inevitably led to confusions, mistakes and Ronald and I began to feel a distinct lack of confidence in the hospital staff.

This was of course a painful time for Ronald, but also a difficult time for me and very worrying for both of us. I was grateful to be able to stay with David and Sue Ramsbotham in their Kensington home while Ronald was in hospital.

I have always thought of Sue and David Ramsbotham as our first 'joint' friends. Marrying later in life and coming from different worlds, Ronald and I initially shared no mutual friends other than my sister, Felicity.

Although Ronald and David had known each other in their student days, they had lost touch. The day after we returned from our honeymoon in September 1978 Ronald was due to lecture to a large group of army chaplains at Bagshot Park. To his delight and surprise David and Sue were in the audience. David had become a colonel in the army and the couple now had two teenage sons. We walked round the grounds together afterwards. The men reminisced while Sue and I discovered what we had in common. The truth was that we had very little. Our only experience we shared was a rural childhood in the North, she in Northumberland and I in Yorkshire.

While my childhood had been happy and I enjoyed our ponies, Sue had hated both. She had married early, become a mother and army officer's wife while I had pursued a career in medicine and married late. Sue's main interests and knowledge were in the arts. I had a huge gap in that area. An unpromising start – we were in many ways complete opposites. Perhaps that's part of why we became close friends – and we do seem to laugh at the same things.

Ronald and David never had any shortage of shared interests from gardening to global security. And indeed David and I found unexpected links. When he enthusiastically told me of the work of Home Start and its potential value for army families, I mentioned that I was one of the trustees of that charity. As the Chief Inspector of Prisons, he was ready to support a Home Start initiative for families stressed by having a parent in prison. As chairman of an NHS hospital trust, he promoted my work on multiple births. Meanwhile Ronald and Sue had lively discussions on political issues or the arts to which I could make little contribution.

And so it was a godsend that I was able to stay so close to Ronald with friends that we had known for over 20 years. Despite the setbacks, Ronald's spirits and appetite soon returned and he was finding hospital incarceration tedious. Luckily there was no shortage of friends eager to entertain him. I soon became the rather grumpy social secretary trying to arrange a timetable for up to five visitors a day. I kept a second telephone in my office with an answerphone bulletin on Ronald and instructions on how to make an appointment to visit him.

My own job was in a busy phase and juggling my work schedule with my new carer and social secretary roles was sometimes not easy. I was surprised how irritable I became. It was the first time I had had to try and combine work and caring and it made me realise how difficult it must be for some of the working mothers (and fathers) of my patients, trying to work while worrying about and looking after a sick child.

I would usually visit Ronald on the way to my own hospital early in the morning and then in the evening on the way back to the Ramsbothams. By then we were both tired and his other visitors had always brought him such exciting delicacies and presents that I couldn't compete. They had also given him much more scintillating conversation than I could. The other problem was that Ronald and I were both upset by some of the faults in his care. I felt impotent to help and sometimes became unreasonably defensive on behalf of my medical colleagues.

As I now look back on all this, I think I should have adopted Ronald's hospital visiting practice. During the three admissions I have had to hospitals for major surgery – two in London and one in Birmingham – Ronald had waited to make sure that I was safely round from the anaesthetic or out of Intensive Care and then, with my encouragement, returned to Herefordshire to prepare the house for my return. It was a much better strategy. We were always very pleased to see each other after the break.

In addition to lapses in his care, the hospital also failed to mention the possibility, let alone prepare Ronald, for what was to become a lifelong handicap and sometimes life-threatening complication resulting from his surgery. Following the removal of glands from the groin, lymph drainage can be interrupted and lymphoedema[5] can develop, which causes permanent swelling of the leg. To drain the lymph the limb has to remain elevated.

Over the years Ronald has become ingenious in coping with his condition. The foldable/portable stool goes everywhere with us and is essential under the dining table, at the cinema, on the train, and in the aeroplane. At theatres we always have to ask for an aisle seat – and at the right end. In bed we have learnt to sleep

---

[5] Lymphoedema is a condition where fluid is retained in a localised area, and is caused by a compromised lymphatic system.

with the end of the mattress raised and his feet tipped up above the level of our heads. Half an hour of leg massage, daily for the first few years and now a few times a week, or sessions with an electric pump, help to drain the leg at the start of the day. A tight, full-length elastic stocking then prevents the leg swelling again.

The other complication of the surgery is that, without lymph glands, the leg becomes much more vulnerable to infection. Out of the blue, about once a year, Ronald develops a form of septicaemia, suddenly starting to shake and vomit. These episodes could be life-threatening but we know now that if he is given large intravenous doses of penicillin immediately, he will recover fully within a few days. Unfortunately fate does not always choose convenient places for him to succumb. A convent in Bahia Salvador in northern Brazil was particularly alarming. Ronald now takes preventive antibiotics during long-haul journeys and I go armed with a battery of penicillin injections for him.

Apart from the inevitable and enduring anxieties about recurrence of his cancer and the lesser, but still real, worries about these frightening infections, there have been a number of ways in which the feel and pattern of our life has had to change.

The most obvious concerns driving. I have never particularly enjoyed it and Ronald had usually taken the wheel when we were travelling together. Returning from evening parties was the only regular exception. Things were now to change. For many months he was entirely dependent on me even for an excursion to the post office and nearest shop in Peterchurch, two miles away. Even now, nine years later, his leg does not allow him more than 30 minutes or so of driving before it becomes uncomfortable and soon distinctly painful.

As a passenger, life was different for him too. Because he has to keep his leg elevated, Ronald always sits in the back of the car. As an inveterate 'backseat driver' by nature, he was now perfectly placed. But neither of us was at ease in our new roles. He felt vulnerable as well as sometimes uncomfortable. In the back seat, especially with a leg up, bumps are more troublesome and braking suddenly becomes much more disconcerting for him.

Thanks to Ronald's daily and ongoing tuition, I now consider myself quite a good and careful driver, but there is clearly still room for improvement and sometimes I am an irritable pupil.

The biggest change in our life due to Ronald's troublesome leg is our wonderful new home. Over nearly 30 years first Ronald and then the two of us together had been gradually enlarging and improving our cottage. Little Reeve had started as a two up, two down cottage on a steep hillside. In 1970 the only taps had been in the kitchen and so was the bath, which had been placed behind a cardboard screen. Over the years our home had acquired two proper bathrooms, a splendid oak-beamed sitting room with gallery, a large third bedroom, a conservatory and the 'Retreat', a large insulated wooden hut with a woodstove, which doubled up as my study and another spare room.

It was perfectly situated in an acre and a half of carefully developed garden, vegetable plots and orchards, reached in its virtual isolation down a peaceful cart track and looking out far across the Golden Valley at the Black Mountains. We loved our home and would have hated to move. But it now had a serious disadvantage. The house was up and down many steps, effectively it was on seven different levels. It was a recipe for disaster for someone with a sometimes painful and rather unsteady leg.

Little Reeve was halfway down this cul-de-sac of a cart track and the only other building was a small cottage, right at the end, another 100 yards beyond us. This other cottage sat under a huge yew tree in five acres of unspoiled pasture and woodland. In it lived Alice Jones, our friend and neighbour for all the years we had spent in Little Reeve, who was now a widow in her late eighties. She had managed valiantly for many years on her own, but a few months before Ronald's operation, she decided to move into a more suitable place in Hereford, nearer to her family.

Alice had been the perfect neighbour and we had been spoilt by the tranquillity down our cart track. We did not want this to change so we had resolved to try and buy Alice's cottage and land to preserve this peace. We had no thoughts beyond that.

Within weeks of learning that our bid had won, after the agonising suspense of a Scottish auction, we also learned that Ronald was to have his operation. Whatever happened, we realised that we could not remain for long at Little Reeve. The message was clear: build a house suitable for him and his leg on our new idyllically placed five acres. It was heaven sent. We would lose none of the advantages of Little Reeve, including our many friendly neighbours, but we would gain an even better view, even greater gardening opportunities and a much more manageable home – if we designed and built it right.

We got straight down to it. Everything began to fall into

place in a wonderful way. At a Christmas party a friend told us of their neighbour, Roderick James, in Devon who built green oak houses. He led a brilliant team of architects and carpenter/joiners in his firm that he had named Carpenter Oak. There was no time to lose. We didn't know how long Ronald would be out of action, so the week before his operation we went down to Devon to meet Roderick and to see examples of his work.

Roderick then visited us to see the five-acre site, which he thought wonderful, and learn about our pattern of life, which he probably thought strange. The essentials of our new house were to be that we took full advantage of one of the loveliest views in England, especially from our bedroom, that it should cater for all eventualities, for either or both of us, and to have a large room for entertaining.

The house had to be wheelchair friendly with our bedroom and Ronald's study on the ground floor and there should be a good-size bedroom with an en suite well away in sound and distance from ours. This would primarily be for the nephews, nieces and godchildren whom we welcomed, and who found our home invaluable for peaceful periods of revision.

This distant room would also be available to convert into a self-contained bedsitter for a carer should the need arise, or for a lodger should one of us be left on their own. At that time there was a serious chance that I might be on my own for many years.

In January 1999 we moved into the first finished room of our new, warm and welcoming home, which we named Quercwm, and on a sun-filled July day that summer we celebrated Ronald's seventieth birthday, his recovery and our new home with a party for relations and close friends.

Even while focusing on Ronald's illness and our house building, there had been no lull in the family cancer saga. In March 1999 I received an email from Bruce Ponder, now Professor, at the Cambridge Cancer Research Group saying they had finally identified a mutation in the BRCA1 gene in our family: 'a deletion of 4 bases designated 3875 del 4'. He thought there was no doubt that this was the 'pathogenic mutation', the abnormal gene, which was causing the predisposition to ovarian cancer in our family. The implication of this discovery was that now anyone in our family who wished it could be tested to see whether or not they had inherited the cancer gene.

Until now none of us had had any way of knowing whether or not we had inherited the gene until it revealed itself as a cancer. All Felicity and I had known was that once Bunny had shown herself to be affected with ovarian cancer then our chances of being one of our family cancer gene carriers had doubled from 25 per cent to 50 per cent as we now knew we had a first-degree relative, our sister, with ovarian cancer, in addition to our grandmother.

At this point no living members of the family had been tested. The gene had been discovered by testing tissues from two members of the family who had died of ovarian cancer.

I had never had any doubt that I wanted to be tested; I went for the obligatory pre-test counselling. For many people this may involve several sessions with a genetic counsellor, someone trained to inform members of families like ours of the implications of being tested, of the reactions we might have to the result whether it be positive or negative, the options that would then be available to us and what actions we might consider taking. Following the test itself the genetic counsellor may be the person who actually gives the result, as they, already knowing the individual, are often in the best position to support them in their inevitable disappointment if they turn out to be a cancer gene carrier and to support them in any further choices they may want to consider. Sometimes their support may be needed for many years to come.

Thanks to all the helpful conversations and correspondence with Bruce Ponder, I had already had a chance to consider all these issues so my visit to the counsellor was brief and I had blood taken for genetic analysis without more ado.

On 17 September 1999, 24 years after Nancy Maguire had first drawn my attention to the cancer in our family, I had a letter from Professor Ponder saying that the test had shown that I *had* inherited the BRCA1 gene mutation that ran in my family.

It is strange how little I remember about my reaction to that news. It certainly caused me no severe or lasting emotional upset. Of course, had the test shown that I was not a cancer gene carrier I am sure I should have been jubilant. But as it was, it was what I had expected and I probably felt a rather weary acceptance. At least the operation to remove my ovaries had been vindicated. Nor did it alter my plan of action. I had already had my ovaries removed and was having regular screening of my breasts.

Professor Ponder discussed the risk for those of us who carry the cancer gene of actually developing cancer of the breast or ovary. He explained that he could only give an estimate based on the average across all the different mutations of the BRCA1 gene and that it was quite likely that different mutations had somewhat different effects. He said that it was also clear that the risk could be modified by other genes as well as by environmental factors, such as taking the contraceptive pill. Despite analysing the largest set of families available, there was still much that was not yet known about what affected the development of the cancers and thus the actual risk to any given individual.

Although I knew that a BRCA1 cancer gene usually gave an increased risk of breast, as well as ovarian, cancer, I was not unduly concerned as there had never been a recorded case of it in our family.

Then on 24 November 1999 Felicity was having her morning shower when she felt a little lump to the side of her left breast. She saw her GP that afternoon who said that although it was probably benign, considering the family history she should see a specialist right away. Very soon a biopsy had shown that the lump was indeed malignant and on 21 December it was removed. Felicity seemed fated to have her operations just before Christmas. A few days later she heard that there was no sign that the cancer had spread to the lymph glands. She would not, therefore, need chemotherapy.

A blood test later confirmed that Felicity too had inherited the family cancer gene. This did not come as a surprise to her. Like me, she had expected a positive result. She remembers the counsellor being on hand, 'all solicitous, and feeling touched by her concern but not needing support'. She was, however, very annoyed as it meant that she was a carrier and her children could thus inherit the gene. With hindsight she feels she should have considered having a double mastectomy there and then. But it did not cross her mind.

Our luck had been bad. All three sisters had turned out to be carriers of the cancer gene and it now looked as if breast cancer was a threat after all.

Felicity was to have a six-week course of 16 doses of radiotherapy. She was also to take Tamoxifen, a drug which was thought to help prevent the spread of the original breast tumour and to avoid the development of other primary tumours.

Her radiotherapy was due to start on 8 March 2000. On the morning of 2 March she was at work when she received a phone call from the school nurse at Oxford High School. Her daughter Alice, now 17 and a lively, articulate girl, had walked out of her mock A-level exams. She was trembling and speechless. Felicity made an emergency appointment with their GP and now recalls:

That afternoon I took Alice to the doctor. Her speech was what he referred to as 'retarded'. He plainly recognised the symptoms of depression right away. She must be taken out of school. She should take no more exams. She should not be left alone. He prescribed medication and made an appointment for her to see a psychiatrist specialising in adolescents. Within days Alice had cut her wrists and a week later she took an overdose. In both cases she told someone immediately and was rushed to hospital. They were cries for help.

My appointments diary during that period makes odd reading. Visits to the radiotherapy department are interspersed with visits to the adolescent psychiatric hospital with Alice. The hospitals were close to each other. It became like a bleak school run.

Not surprisingly Felicity remembers little of her own health and treatments during this time as all her concern, and indeed that of the family, was focused on Alice, who we had known as a bright independent teenager expected to do well in her A levels, take a gap year abroad, go to university, and so on. Now she was profoundly depressed. She turned 18 by June 2000, so that when she actually became psychotic she was admitted to an adult psychiatric hospital.

By April 2000 when Felicity was coming to the end of her radiotherapy treatment I felt obliged to think about the future, of the preventive measures I should be considering, and of the next generation. Ronald and I again went off to see Professor Ponder. First he discussed my own risk of breast cancer and said that on the information currently available I had a 30 per cent chance of developing breast cancer by the age of 80, but the chance of dying from it was considerably less. As to what I could do about it, my options were to continue screening with regular mammograms or have a preventive bilateral mastectomy. Currently, he said, there was no drug proven to reduce the risk, although a trial of Tamoxifen was in progress.

We talked about a mastectomy, which would reduce the risk of breast cancer by about 95 per cent but not remove the risk altogether. The last few percentages of protection depended on the extent of the surgery. A balance had to be struck between the possible side effects of extensive surgery such as permanently swollen arms from lymphoedema and the almost complete removal of any risk of cancer. That could only be decided by discussion between a specialist surgeon and myself.

I concluded that I would prefer to take the risk of developing cancer than lose my breasts but would have very regular ultrasound screening to give the best chance of any cancer being caught early and treated successfully.

Professor Ponder and his team have always been as

interested in the emotional and psychological impact of the threat of cancer on individuals and their families as they have in the science of its genetic causes, prevention and treatment. I was therefore keen to discuss the likely impact on the next generation, my five nieces and nephews who were now aged between 12 and 18.

Professor Ponder said that the guiding principles in telling young people were that they should be fully able to take their own decisions, in due course, about what they want to do – in particular about having a genetic test; and that, at the present time, as teenagers, there was no preventive action of any kind that one would recommend even if they were known to carry the cancer gene. So they were not missing out by not knowing.

He said that the choice of when to talk to them about it would depend on a variety of things including how we communicated as a family, what the attitudes of the young were likely to be, whether they were already asking questions, whether they were likely to hear about it from other members of the family, and so on. This was a judgement, he said, that only we, the family members, can make.

However he did add a cautionary note:

It is often children who have seen the death of a parent while they were in their teenage years who are most upset by the whole business of familial cancer; and second that it is a pity if receiving this information at a time when they are making important life choices – about marriage or a career – leads young people into what one might call an unnecessarily defensive attitude.

He also mentioned his team's approach to families on their

register as new information came available. This was of course relevant to my own wider family, some of whom I was in touch with, but the majority of whom I had never met or had lost touch with many years before. He continued by saying:

> We are already contacting those members of the family who have 'signed up' for our research studies, where part of the deal was that we would get back to them in due course when we had some potentially useful information. The terms in which we contact them are just that: that we have some information, and they might like to contact us so that we can discuss with them whether they would like to know more. We are careful not to tell them at the outset that we know what the mutation is in the family or to come across with possibly threatening information which they may decide they do not want to hear. . .
>
> I think it would be useful and appropriate if you were to indicate to branches of the family who might not know about it, that this information is potentially available. . .
>
> I would urge you to remember that as a doctor familiar with these things, and as an individual who has confronted the problem and taken positive action about it, you may well have a different outlook from others of your relatives. Once you have given them information, it is like a pill, you cannot take it back. So do be circumspect!

I told my nephews' and nieces' parents, Felicity, Alex and Rob, what Professor Ponder had said. We all agreed that there was no need to worry the children with any of this information at least until their mid-twenties. At the same time we would keep ourselves informed so that we were ready to answer any questions should they ask them. I was surprised that not one of these five bright teenagers had so far questioned the very obvious cancer in our family, let alone whether it had any implications for them. Perhaps they feared the answer so did not want to ask, perhaps they were protecting their parents. Perhaps the most likely explanation is that most teenagers are so preoccupied with their day-to-day lives that a potential problem so far in the future is beyond their horizon.

By May 2000 Felicity had finished her treatment and there was a very good chance that it had been caught early enough to avoid a recurrence. Cancer was no longer our main concern, particularly in Felicity's family. A much greater one was Alice's illness. In August she had jumped off the roof of her home breaking her back in three places. While she recovered well following surgery, her depression continued. And by Christmas she was manic. It looked as if she had inherited her grandmother's bipolar disorder – manic depression.

There followed a dreadful year. But by the summer of 2002 Alice was much better. She had been accepted to do an Art Foundation Course in Banbury. She started on 9 September. That same day Felicity discovered another lump – now in the other breast. This time she knew the routine. She regarded her surgeon, Miss Clarke, as a friend.

When she delivered the bad news that the tumour was malignant she gave me a memorable hug. She said that this recurrence showed that my gene was 'expressing itself'. She need say no more. Without even looking at Alex I looked down at my bosoms and said I regarded them as time bombs and wanted them both off at her earliest convenience. She said that before that she would like me to have other tests to see if the cancer was elsewhere in my body. If it had spread then clearly our plan of action would be different. I saw her point. Having my breasts off if there was cancer elsewhere would be like shutting the stable door when the horse has bolted. But while she booked the tests we provisionally booked me in for the double mastectomy on 22 October – conveniently after my annual week at the Frankfurt Book Fair.

Bone scans and X-rays of her chest and abdomen showed no signs of cancer in the rest of her body. This was another primary cancer. Felicity would go ahead with a double mastectomy.

I think both Felicity and I have probably inherited a certain pragmatism and decisiveness from our father. Through all the various stages of our illnesses, I don't remember either of us spending much time trying to decide what to do next either in terms of prevention or treatment. If anything, my decision making tends to be too impetuous. Although appreciating the value of counselling, it is not something for which I have ever felt the need in order to make a decision.

Felicity is equally decisive. She says:

I did not much mind the thought of losing my breasts because I was so determined to eliminate further chances of cancer. But I did assume that I would have reconstruction – and indeed spent some time photographing my bosoms to enlighten the plastic surgeon who would be reconstructing them. . . Miss Clarke had advised against reconstruction in the same operation as removing my breasts as she said that if I had to have radiotherapy later – which it turned out that I did – radiation could have an unsatisfactory 'cosmetic effect' on re-constructed breasts.

Once they were removed I was surprised how little I minded. I remember my childhood friend Tricia visiting me in hospital just after my dressings were removed. 'Do you want to look?' I said and she said 'Aaah, how sweet.' And, I suppose because I am so small, there was indeed something childlike about my new look.

Tests taken during the operation showed that there had this time been some cancer spread into the lymph glands in her armpit. This meant that once she had recovered from the operation and her wounds had healed Felicity would have a course of chemotherapy followed by another of radiotherapy.

She went ahead, losing her hair in the process and wearing a succession of elegant turbans.

There is little new to say about the chemotherapy, which I hated and made me feel weak and lose my hair. The radiotherapy I found – as before – strangely peaceful, lying there still and alone in that huge room while the enormous machine that looked like something out of *Star Wars* hovered above me in the half light making its clicking and whirring noises, radiating away. After my first session I was putting my clothes back on and a small Indian nurse tapped me on the arm. 'It's Mrs Duncan, isn't it?' she said. 'I remember you from last time. I hope you don't mind me asking but how is your daughter?' I was speechless. It had been nearly three years since she had treated me. She had seen literally thousands of patients in the intervening time. But she had remembered my anxiety. She was the very best kind of nurse. I cannot tell you how moved I was.

In fact Felicity never had her breast reconstructions. Four years later she reflected on why she changed her mind:

I think my main reason is that I so hate being 'post-operative'. The doctors tend to say you will feel normal in, say, six months. Everybody reacts differently but in my experience it was well over a year. After a year I feel okay and just think the reason I am tired is that I am getting a bit older. Then suddenly at nearer 18 months I realise I am my energetic self again. With three cancers and one oophorectomy with hysterectomy I have been post-operative four times. I now wanted to get back to my family and on with my life; the thought of willingly electing to have major surgery for the fifth time in eight years – and just for the look of it – seemed plain silly.

6

More Preventive Measures

WHEN, IN OCTOBER 2002, Felicity found a second lump in her breast, I suddenly realised I could no longer live with my own risk of breast cancer. Up until then I had been happy to continue with annual mammograms. Now the threat was too great. I wanted to be rid of my potentially deadly appendages.

I didn't hesitate. Of course electing to have such an operation must be a much tougher decision for someone in her thirties, or for someone who was not yet in a long-term relationship or who had not had children. For me it was not difficult. I just wanted to do everything I could to avoid cancer.

I know that many people are horrified at the idea of removing two healthy breasts. Some feel it challenges their femininity, their very identity. For many people the thought of the change in their body image is devastating. My body image has never been of great pride to me, and my breasts were not something for which I had a particular affection. Perhaps I resented them for having never performed their main function: they had given me no rewarding memories of breastfeeding.

At the time I gave myself other arguments. As the only sister, at that point, free from cancer, I had a duty to the next generation to remain healthy if I possibly could. I probably wasn't honest to myself – I expect the main reason was that I wanted to do all I could to go on living this rich life.

But I was concerned how Ronald might respond to the suggestion. I need not have worried. He agreed immediately. As with the removal of my womb and ovaries, 10 years before, his only concern was that I should live a healthy life for as long as possible. He seemed less concerned than I did as to the extent that artificial breasts would affect our physical relationship.

Having made the decision, I then felt awkward about telling Felicity. It seemed heartless to be thinking of removing two healthy breasts when she had had no option but to suffer the physical and emotional trauma of losing hers to cancer. But before I got round to telling her, Felicity in her usual straight-forwardly pragmatic way actually asked me if I was going to have a preventive mastectomy. She clearly thought that was the sensible thing to do. In retrospect I am surprised that I hadn't considered the option more seriously three years before, when Felicity's first malignant breast tumour was diagnosed.

My next concern was the younger generation. Up until then, there was no reason for my nieces to have made any connection between their mother's and their aunt's cancer with anyone else in the family. If I now had such drastic surgery they were bound to ask why I was taking such an extreme step. I therefore, for the first time, decided on secrecy.

The need to protect the girls influenced my decision as to whether to have my breasts reconstructed. The alternative, that of remaining flat-chested with the help of artificial breasts as Felicity had done, was clearly the simplest route – and, as it turned out, would have been much less troublesome in the long run.

I know that many people who have had a mastectomy for cancer feel mutilated, angry and very unhappy with their now flat, scarred, but otherwise featureless chest. I was not worried about that so long as I could look normal in public. I would have been quite content to use silicone prostheses that fit into the extensive range of attractive pocketed bras and high cut swimming costumes advertised in the Nicola Jane catalogue, which is targeted at women who have lost their breasts through cancer or other surgery.

However, a flat chest would be almost impossible to conceal from my nieces. We holiday together, often sharing a changing room and sometimes a bedroom. A sudden erasure of prominent parts would have provoked both surprise and questions. This was probably my main reason for deciding to have some form of artificial breast. But it turned out to be a decision with a higher price to pay in worry, money and discomfort than I had expected.

I was unlikely to be able to have two healthy breasts removed under the NHS, let alone any form of reconstruction. And the procedure would certainly not be carried out by a surgeon of my choice. I therefore sought advice and was recommended an internationally renowned breast surgeon together with his colleague, a plastic surgeon. These two, who worked privately, explained what was involved and discussed whether the reconstruction of my breasts should consist of silicone implants or tissue transplanted from other parts of my body. The implants were a less invasive operation and would still allow a tissue transplant in the future if needed.

The surgeons also explained that my nipples would be removed because of the risk of cancer developing in their ducts but that imitations could be created some months after the original operation either from a little 'button' of skin or by tattooing.

I was given a booklet which explained that 'reconstructed breasts are a little firmer and more erect, like young women's breasts' rather than those of older women who 'often have slightly drooping breasts'. It then went on to say that in those women having a single mastectomy it may be advisable to have the other one lifted slightly or enlarged. I could see that those single-breast people had even more decisions to make than I had – although their decision would be simpler when it came to the nipples.

Both the surgeons respected my reasons for wanting my breasts removed and agreed to perform the operations. After discussing the various options and operations on offer, we decided that I should have both breasts removed and silicone implants inserted during a single operation. I should expect four days or so in hospital and should be pretty well back to normal activities within three weeks. I was glad neither surgeon suggested I needed to see a counsellor. I had made the decision and did not want it made harder by discussing the possible emotional and physical complications and nothing was going to change my mind now.

I was given time to ask questions and I am sure could have met other women who had undergone a mastectomy and reconstruction, if I had requested it. But I was so impatient to get rid of my breasts that I didn't take advantage of those opportunities. I came to regret that. It would not have affected my decision but I might have been better prepared for some of the difficulties that lay ahead: the physical discomforts, the restriction of movement and activities. All of which resolved in the end but took a long time to do so.

The plastic surgeon carefully noted my present breasts and I was asked if I wanted any change in their size. As I was used to myself as I was, I asked for them to stay the same. This was probably a mistake. If I had chosen smaller implants, it might have been less strain on my not-so-young muscle and skin tissue.

In November 2002 I was admitted to the private ward of a London hospital and had bilateral mastectomies and what are termed anatomical implant reconstructions. That is to say that once the breast tissue had been removed, a silicone implant was inserted in its place under the muscle and skin. 'Anatomical' refers to the shape of the implant which is shaped more like a teardrop rather than a sphere in order to follow the body's lines. They are designed to give the breasts a more natural shape.

After I came out of surgery I was told that the operation had gone well and I was making a good recovery.

However nothing had prepared me for the iron grip that held my chest – or so it felt. I believe some people have one breast removed at a time. I can understand why. It is hard having tubes coming out of both sides of you and knowing that it will be equally painful whichever way you turn. Nevertheless I was out of bed on the first day after my operation and home on the sixth.

Going home meant a train journey of 150 miles but Ronald came to help and it was done in as much comfort as the train could provide. Had I remained in London I would probably have gone for daily inspection of my wound at the hospital. As it was, my own family doctor and the community nurse gave me daily and careful attention. However, none of us wanted to disturb the dressings and it was only after a few days that it became apparent that all was not well beneath the bandages on the left side. A peek of bright red skin was visible.

Initially we thought this was an infection developing and I was given antibiotics. Although I never became feverish my breast continued to look most unhappy. Two weeks after my operation I was readmitted to hospital in London for a course of intravenous antibiotics. Despite this, my left breast remained swollen and tense before suddenly expelling a large amount of fluid. The fluid was thought to be the result of breakdown of the fatty tissue in the left breast flap. Having got rid of the fluid, I felt more comfortable but it was clear that there was still a problem.

At this point I was despondent. Had I made the biggest mistake of my life? Was I risking my life rather than saving it? Realistically, however worrisome the condition of my breasts was, my life was not in danger. I was just seriously disconcerted that my plans for a short secretive operation had gone so very wrong. No longer was it possible for friends to remain in ignorance. I was readmitted to hospital and was clearly not my usual healthy self.

Furthermore an important trip to Australia was now in jeopardy. I had been invited to give a lecture in Melbourne in early February. Ronald was to accompany me and we had planned to see friends and to have a holiday while we were over there. I clearly couldn't travel in this state; time was running out.

Meanwhile my father was critically ill in Yorkshire, so as soon as I could get back on to oral antibiotics I took the 250-mile train journey to visit him. A week later he and I were both feeling better, however, there was now an ominous hole at the bottom of the scar on my left breast.

If the hole was left unsealed there would be a continuing risk of infection but the skin round the hole was now too fragile to sew up again. There seemed no alternative but to remove the implant and to insert a much smaller one, one that could gradually be inflated with small volumes of saline at intervals over the next few months through a valve under my arm attached to the implant.

My surgeon agreed that I should go home and enjoy Christmas and the New Year and allow everything to settle down. On 6 January 2003 I was readmitted for another operation under general anaesthetic during which the original implant was replaced by a 'deflated expander prosthesis' and valve. For many weeks it gave me a shock to feel this pebble as big as a Brazil nut under my arm every time I showered. Now I rarely notice it.

Twenty-one days after the second operation I set off for Australia. This had remained my goal over the previous two months. Sunbathing and swimming in an Australian January seemed the perfect recipe for convalescence. My doctors agreed.

Although by now the iron grip around my chest had lessened, it was still quite strong, which meant that the flight was not comfortable, and 18 hours of relative immobility certainly didn't help. But equipped with my smart new high-cut Nicola Jane costume, the thought of a gentle swim had become increasingly attractive as we approached Singapore, where we were to have a 48-hour stopover before continuing to Australia.

A shock awaited me. As I eagerly dipped into the pool, I found I was quite unable to swim. Not only was a breast-stroke painful but my strokes were too weak to keep me afloat. I can rarely remember feeling as disappointed as I did then. I felt like a child who had missed the outing of a lifetime. After a lot of hard work I managed to swim a short distance with a sort of doggy paddle. Gradually over the next few weeks I relearnt a tentative breast-stroke.

By the end of February I was back in England after our holiday. My scar had healed well and I was feeling much more cheerful and comfortable. There were still major inconveniences like having to sleep on my back. I took a long time to adjust to this, but luckily the practice run came in handy for the much bigger operation that was to follow a few years later.

There were more shocks followed by adaptations to be made along the way – not just to do with swimming. When I first tried to play tennis again, my arm hit an obstacle as I tried to throw the ball up to serve. I literally bumped into myself. Firmer than before and jutting out sideways my left breast interrupted my throw. Kate Dooher in her book *I've Got Cancer But Cancer Hasn't Got Me*, describes a similar more embarrassing experience when she tried to raise her glass to give a toast. The contents went flying as her rising arm hit a protrusion.

On my next visit to the clinic, we agreed that it was time to reduce the very marked lopsidedness of my breasts and to start inflating the left one. The surgeon began very gently with only 20 millilitres of saline. By mid-April I had had 120 millilitres injected. By mid-June I reached the total of 180 millilitres.

At this point we needed to discuss the reconstruction of my

nipples. The best of reconstructed breasts are ugly when nipple-less. And mine were no exception. They had not yet settled and looked to me like two thick pancakes or perhaps more accurately failed sponge cakes. They badly needed adornment.

My plastic surgeon was wary of interfering in any way with the still fragile skin on my left breast. I therefore happily accepted his suggestion of tattooed nipples.

There was a nurse in the plastic surgery unit who specialised in this craft. With the skill and dedication of an artist she explained how the tattooing was done and the decisions that had to be made.

I regretted that I had not studied my nipples more carefully in the past. Just as I am bad at noticing or remembering the colour of people's eyes, I realised that I had no idea what colour my nipples had been. Clearly this is where those with a single mastectomy are at an advantage as they have a colour match close by.

I was handed a card that reminded me of the one presented by the hairdresser when choosing the next tint. The nurse's own enthusiasm made me feel I should have stronger views. As it was I was just grateful for any advice she gave me and chose a colour accordingly. I had two sessions of tattooing. It was an odd sensation but not painful and I was delighted with the result. I felt transformed. Ronald, who had been amazingly restrained in not commenting before, clearly thought there had been a significant improvement.

Even without the various setbacks, at 60 and 74 I doubt that our sex life would have been a page-turner. Indeed it probably never had been. Sex had always been a very happy, straight-forward, vital and yet unadventurous part of our life.

It had inevitably been challenged at times but had survived the earlier struggles with remarkable fortitude. To enhance our chances of conception, for many months Ronald had gallantly performed (even, when necessary, into little plastic pots) and abstained to order.

My hysterectomy caused only a minor setback to our sex life, which resumed straightforwardly after a short convalescence. Ronald's major surgery undoubtedly proved a bigger hurdle. The foot-up angle of his side of our bed didn't help matters. Nor has the need for a long bolster to separate us at times, to avoid risking damage to our various tender parts following surgery to his leg or my abdomen and breasts. I have always returned from hospital straight to the marital bed. The few weeks when Ronald's wound was infected and he had an MRSA infection was the only time at home when we could not sleep together.

As our sex life became more restricted, our need for, and pleasure from, physical contact had, if anything, increased. Hugging, cuddling and handholding are crucially important to us and have often been a lifeline for me.

My very real fears of the effect on Ronald of my mastectomy were unfounded. I would have understood, however sadly, if he had been unable to touch my body with the affection he had in the past. Either through love or generosity or both, as soon as the tenderness had settled he tried stroking my breasts. What neither of us had reckoned on was that this was now the least erotic part of my body. It was numb. He might as well have stroked my cheek on the way home from a dentist's local anaesthetic.

But luckily there were other outlets. Ever since our wooing days, handholding has been a natural part of our life, whether in church, at concerts or just walking. By now we must have looked like one of the Derby and Joan couples that we had probably watched with condescending amusement in our earlier days. Unlike most couples, our own handholding habits have never been broken by smaller hands competing for ours, and our physical proximity has never been interrupted by a child when sitting in an aeroplane, watching a film or listening to a sermon.

Physical contact, touch, became increasingly important through the trials to come.

7

My Father's Cancer and Two Deaths

IT IS AUGUST 2003 on a hot fine evening in the mountains of
Andalusia. Twenty-three of us are sitting around a table on the
terrace of a *palacete* (a Spanish type of mansion) celebrating my
father's ninetieth birthday.

The whole family is gathered here. Along with my father and
his two surviving children, Felicity and myself, are my stepmother, Cynthia, and her four children. All our partners are
there too, together with all 11 grandchildren. Ages range from
my father's 90 years down to my five-year-old twin nieces. The
only ones missing are Bunny and Rob.

The family has come together at a particularly happy time.
Everyone is healthy. Behind us are illnesses and bereavements,
but they are in the past. At this golden Spanish sunset, life is
particularly good. It is time for celebration, and celebrate we do.
My father, although frail, is in buoyant spirits and, with a
politician's skill, delivers a note-free speech praising the talents
of each of his grandchildren in turn. My stepmother, Cynthia,
gave us a memorable recitation of 'Albert and the Lion'.

A good Spanish dinner is followed by entertainment from
the grandchildren, mostly skits at the expense of the adults,

some daringly candid. And the evening ends with an elaborate song and dance presentation to my father of one of his favourite tunes, 'You're the Cream in my Coffee'.

Such gatherings have become rare as the family was usually scattered between London, New York, La Rochelle, Oxford, Yorkshire and Herefordshire, so on this beautiful summer's evening we welcome the chance to be together. The diversity of interests and occupations means that there is no shortage of conversation or debate. There is a diversity of activities too for when we're not gathered around the family table: mountain walking, tennis, swimming, painting, poetry writing, photography, ping-pong, sightseeing, trips to the local market and card games. A casual onlooker could be forgiven for envying such an idyllic scene of family happiness, prosperity and fun.

But that was 2003. The next two years were to be very different.

For the past three years my father had known that he had cancer of the prostate. The BRCA1 cancer gene that we three daughters, and therefore also our father, carried could have been the cause. On the other hand, prostate cancer in general is not uncommon in older men.

My father had confided in me, as his only medically qualified daughter, when his cancer was first diagnosed. Otherwise, he had told no one else except Cynthia. I admired their strength and self-sufficiency in carrying such a burden on their own, something Ronald and I could never have done. Nor should we have wanted to: we were unapologetically dependent on the support of our friends.

But illness was alien to both my father and stepmother. They had always been remarkably fit for their age and neither had previously had any serious illnesses or debility. Both had looked much younger than their years and Cynthia had retained a figure and elegance that were the envy of those of us in the younger generation. My father played golf at least weekly until his late eighties and Cynthia was still beating her children and grandchildren on the tennis court well into her ninth decade. Their energy as a couple put the rest of us to shame. They would think nothing of helping at the village fete in Yorkshire one afternoon, giving a dinner party in the evening and driving to a Sunday lunch in Oxford or London the next day.

They had long had a rule that they would only discuss health matters on Fridays. This was not difficult to keep for most of their married life but my father kept it up until his last year – a remarkable feat of fortitude and restraint for someone who was in almost constant pain for several years.

It was only when he had a serious relapse early in 2003 and looked as if he might die that I persuaded him to tell Felicity and his stepchildren about his cancer; and also to tell Pat and Jack Woodhead and Sue Barnes who were key members of the Park Farm household. Otherwise, apart from his immediate family and medical carers, there were very few, if any, others who knew about his illness. People were left to assume he was just dying of 'old age'. He was by then in his ninetieth year.

Pat and Jack Woodhead had arrived at Park Farm with their three young sons soon after my father and Cynthia married in 1971. Pat was the housekeeper while Jack looked after the garden and drove anyone in need. Sue later joined to help Pat. They lived in the two cottages on the farm. All three were devoted to my father and he regarded them as part of our family. Without their constant help it would never have been possible to nurse him to the end at home; in fact there was no need for any outside nursing help. It was his fervent hope that he could die in his own bed in the beautiful room that he and my mother had designed, which looked out on the Yorkshire Wolds, his parliamentary constituency for so many years. And this he did.

Over the years, I would see my father during his frequent visits to London but rarely visited him in Yorkshire. During the last years, however, as he became confined to Yorkshire, I started going up more often and during the last year alternated fortnightly with Felicity for a midweek visit. It suited everyone well. My father hated the thought of Cynthia, so used to an active life, having to be continually tied at home when she had lots to do and grandchildren to care for in London. Meanwhile Felicity and I enjoyed the chance to spend time alone with our father, reminiscing for hours about our happy childhood in this same house. Cynthia would then return armed with messages and stories from his many friends in the South.

It was a time of great nostalgia and my father revelled in it too.

He also prepared us for his death with great efficiency. He had always been a very orderly person and was determined that both his illness and death should cause us as few problems as possible. He continued to care for himself with stoicism and grit. For someone who had rarely even taken an aspirin, he managed his 16 pills a day with remarkable efficiency and independence. It was only towards the end that I was allowed to help by fortnightly loading ingenious plastic boxes that had slots for the various pills for each part of a given day.

He retained his dignity and sense of humour to the end. Perhaps his experiences of the extremes of hardship in the fierce heat of North Africa and the freezing cold of the Italian campaigns had taught him how to bear prolonged discomfort and pain in a way that most of us never dream of. He persisted with activities long after most would have given up. He would never consider moving to a downstairs room, preferring to struggle up and down the stairs with chairs strategically placed at the two bends for him to rest between stages.

About death he was entirely philosophical and practical. Throughout his life he had always been early for engagements. I have sat in many a lay-by with him having arrived too early for a meeting or party. He was always packed ahead of time. As he had been in life, so he was when preparing for his death. Years before, as he entered his eighties – and was in excellent health – he had already made what he considered the necessary detailed preparations for his death.

His filing cabinet had been pruned to a bare minimum and divided in two. The bottom drawer contained his day-to-day business, all of which could be discarded immediately after his death. The top drawer contained clearly labelled files with papers that might be relevant to the sorting of his estate and the tidying of any other outstanding matters. The filing cabinet was periodically reviewed and repruned, and a list of essential information and relevant names and addresses was updated annually.

As his eldest child, I was given regular conducted tours of his study. He took great pains to introduce me to people who would be able to help in the sorting of his estate and his affairs, as well as the sale of our family home and its 200 acres of farmland and woods. We had expeditions to meet a solicitor, accountant, friendly land agents, farming consultants, experts on shooting rights, a world of which I knew little.

A leader by nature and a commander by experience, it required unusual restraint on my father's part not to instruct me in actions to be taken after his death. He restricted himself to gentle guidance, for which later I was immensely grateful. I was deeply grateful too that we could always talk so openly about his dying and death. He discussed the process in the same pragmatic way as he might have explored plans for his next journey. When he first broached the subject he was anxious to learn about the most likely medical scenarios: sudden death from a brain haemorrhage; a slow decline as the cancer took over; or a relatively rapid terminal illness with an overwhelming infection.

I am sure my medical background allowed him to discuss his concerns more openly than he would otherwise have done and I felt privileged and happy to be able to help him. Although there had always been deep love and respect between us, there had also been some reserve. We were very dissimilar and some of my interests he had no wish to share. Self-analysis was foreign to him and terms such as 'the unconscious' were utterly alien.

Two of his daughters, as a doctor and priest, were in different ways professionally involved with counselling. My father had always made it clear that this was a mystery to him and, by implication at least, not the area of our work that he most admired. This attitude was reinforced by his only personal experience in the field. On one journey from London to York his golf clubs were stolen. On reporting this at the station in

York, the staff promised to do all they could to retrieve them. The following day my father eagerly took a telephone call from British Rail only to be greeted by a soothing voice enquiring how he was feeling about his 'loss' and offering a telephone number for further support should he feel the need!

But now he was able to talk of his feelings perhaps for the first time, of some of his regrets, of his many happinesses and of his worries. He was naturally very concerned for Cynthia. He was also worried for Pat and Jack who he feared might have to move from their cottage on our farm. During these talks with my father I realised, not for the first time, how precious a time the last months and days of life can be for both the dying and their loved ones. And with sadness, I think of how many of us never have those opportunities. Sometimes this is because the death is sudden and unexpected. But often it is because neither the dying person nor those with them can penetrate the reserve from which we all suffer to some extent.

I treasure the memories of those last weeks with my father when we got to know each other, in some ways for the first time. He had only one fear: losing his independence and becoming a burden to others. I also knew that he would hate not to be in command, at least of himself. When a minor stroke impeded his speech he eagerly embarked, already very frail, on exercises provided by the speech therapist. When every step was an effort he would still set off on his daily walk. He valiantly stayed in command of his body and his mind right until the last week.

My father rarely asked for any help but the one way in which I could give him pleasure was by body massage. I have read so often, and personally witnessed, the value of this physical contact to the very ill. Not only can it gently soothe the aches and pains of the bedridden, but the touch itself can both comfort and reassure someone feeling disheartened, even ashamed, by their physical deterioration. Those patients who are not by nature comfortable with physical contact from relative strangers can often accept gratefully the offer of a 'massage'.

My father was closely involved with the life of every one of his 11 grandchildren. He kept in active touch with them all. He realised that third-millennium teenagers were unlikely to be letter writers, so, at 87, he had learnt to type, to email and to study websites. A lively correspondence followed with gap-year grandchildren as far flung as Pakistan and Ecuador. He would proudly download grandson Zafar's weekly contribution to Pakistan's *Friday Times*.

Every one of the grandchildren managed to visit their grandfather during the last weeks of his life. They all, except perhaps the six-year-olds, knew that it was probably the last time they would see him. He would prepare himself for each and discuss their current project or plan with them. Natasha sang songs with him; Alice arrived back from Ecuador just in time and was driven straight up to Yorkshire. As Felicity wrote:

When we tiptoed into my father's bedroom his eyes were closed. He looked dead. But then he boomed 'Alice my darling'. The *Encyclopaedia Britannica* was on the bed, open at Ecuador. He had been mugging up. I left them together. They both knew it was the last time that they would meet.

Catherine, then 16, discussed her plan to visit Peru where he had led a parliamentary delegation 50 years before. She later recalled that last visit to her grandfather in a poem:

'See You Later'

I remember when I saw you last. . .
How I tiptoed through the stifled air
Feeling like a trespasser, prying,
Into a private, ugly world.
Your booming welcome and easy cheer, broke the spell,
And as before
Made all seem well.
I knew you were dying. . . and yet,
When we got talking. . . so easy to forget.
You told me an old story. . .
The Order of Peru,
And the excited words, keen to please,
Had the same enchanting quality,
Like a favourite song heard anew.

I could hardly deserve such interest, as always, in me,
Your eyes wide alert, attention to arrest,
Eagerly discussing future plans and past success.
There was the book you gave me. . . which you read once
It reads. . . With love. . . from Gran and Grandpa
To celebrate all those stars ***. . .

That said the most.

I felt so happy. . . and so sad
I longed to just hug you. . .
Perhaps I wish I had,
But that was not your style.

So I kissed your papery cheeks
And squeezed your shaking hands,
Lovely to see you. . . see you soon
No reply. You just smiled and waved.

I'll see you in another life then.

In those last three years, although his activities became steadily curtailed, his spirit and sense of fun were unquenched. In his last month he was still having lively discussions with friends from his days in politics. During the last week, by now weak and sleeping much of the time, Pat, Jack and I warned him that we were going to hoover and tidy his bedroom. He appeared to be unconscious throughout. When carefully tucked in with sparkling clean sheets, I gently told him that all was now in order. He could rest in peace. He whispered back, 'Let's have a bottle of champagne with Pat and Jack first.'

By his last two days, he was ready to die and was impatient to do so. We discussed the best way to tackle this. I suggested that he should now just rest peacefully back, stop talking and try to sleep. 'But perhaps,' I tentatively suggested, 'you might like to say goodbye to Cynthia first.'

'I've said goodbye to her 18 times.'

Our laughter and tears were intermingled during these last days.

The final hours were peaceful and he died, as planned, in his own bed. It was in the early hours of 11 October 2004 with Cynthia by his side, and Felicity and me in the next room.

Three days later a service was held in a quiet crematorium high on the Yorkshire Wolds. Just family and, of course, Pat,

Jack and Sue. The organist was a retired vicar known best for his jazz playing – so we went in to 'Old Man River' and came out to his favourite 'You're the Cream in my Coffee'. The service was taken by John Allen, a close friend and the retired Provost of Wakefield. Bunny's daughter Catherine bravely read a poem and the eldest grandchild, Patrick, the lesson. The rest of us sang vigorously and wept. We prayed for Bunny too.

The family then dispersed, leaving my stepsister Annie to be with Cynthia at Park Farm while the rest of us picked up the pieces of our temporarily disrupted lives. The next few weeks were spent in the usual arrangements following any death. The letters flooded in bringing comfort, tears and laughter to Cynthia, Felicity and me.

But soon we had to get down to organising the thanksgiving service, which took on the scale of a military operation. My father had been adamant that it should be in his own parish church with his friends from Sawdon and Brompton, where he had lived for over 50 years. He did not want it to be in London. 'Anyway,' he said, 'at my age not many people will come and I don't want it to be a flop!' Little did he realise how much more straightforward for us it would have been to have held it, like many politicians' families, at St Margaret's, Westminster.

The service was to be on Friday 26 November 2004. The weekend before, preparations were nearly complete. The grandchildren were practising their various roles and I was rehearsing my tribute. I had popped back to Herefordshire for a few days. At 4am that Monday morning, the telephone rang. We were used to such disturbances – before the email era we often got faxes from Australia. This time, it was not a fax, but Felicity. Quietly she said 'Alice has died.' Her lovely

22-year-old daughter had taken her own life. As Felicity later wrote:

> On November 21 2004 my daughter Alice, a student at Glasgow School of Art, told her flatmate that she would not after all go out to get some supper with him but felt like taking an early night. She would go to bed with her book. When she was alone she put a plastic bag over her head, secured it very tightly and took her life. The disease [bipolar disorder] from which she had suffered before had returned and would return again. She did not like what she saw ahead.
>
> *Guardian* 22 April 2006

Of course we were all shattered by the news. Although I felt terribly shocked – the last time I had seen Alice she had been so happy and enthusiastic – I was not incredulous. I knew from the many sad years with my mother, how devastating and rapidly changing this cruel disease can be.

Alex, Felicity, Max and Ben went straight up to Glasgow. Led by their courage we knew we had no choice but to go through with our plans for my father's thanksgiving service. Some people expected us to cancel it; Alice would have hated us to do that. She had prepared these words to say at the service. They were found among her possessions after she died:

> I'd known for a long time, we all had, that he was leaving us soon. So you try, at least, to prepare yourself. I thought of everything he'd done for me, said to me, meant to me. How he'd loved us – individually, unconditionally. How proud he was of us – individually, unconditionally. You don't feel worthy of it, but

feel a better person because of it. Yet you can't really prepare yourself. I've never lost a grandfather before – his role is unique. Watching over you your whole life. Questioning, advising, caring, asking after you – always needing to know that you are all right. Loving you so closely yet letting you grow independently.

So we went ahead with no changes other than Alice's piece being beautifully read by her brother Max and a special prayer for her said by her cousin Lizzie, and a word in my tribute.

I ended the tribute to my father:

> In his long life my father taught his children and grandchildren many lessons that we shall treasure. Now he has taught us perhaps the most important one of all, how to die. How to die without fear but with love. With humour, with dignity. And with a deep faith that all would be well. All will be well.

Every member of the family had gathered in Yorkshire for the thanksgiving service.

Nearly all of us met again two weeks later in Kidlington for Alice's funeral.

It was an extraordinary occasion – the church was packed with people of all ages, including a group of student friends from Glasgow and her tutor. Tributes were given by her father, her brother Max, her cousin Gina, her best friend Ros and me. There was little need to remind friends of the extraordinary courage, talent and suffering of a beautiful girl who had been loved by so many. We then sang hymns in the graveyard while her father, brothers and friends gradually filled her grave.

At the wake afterwards many friends spoke of their own

memories of Alice. Of the Alice described by her tutor as 'kind, alert, witty, cheeky, warm, intelligent and very talented'. Her godmother and godfather suggested that a collection of her remarkable photographs be made into a book. This has now been produced[6] and includes some of her writings. The most poignant perhaps is the following poem:

'Response to Cynicism'

Some work comes from sadness
Other springs from joy.
Angst, also, can produce the heartbreak blow
Needed to create

Sometimes the best way is to sit on a bench
        and watch the rain fall
And so it makes me wonder, now and again,
How anyone can be cynical
Of emotions as pure as these.

March 2004

The next few months were sad for all of us, devastating for Alice's family. Deaths in the autumn inevitably make Christmas difficult to cope with. Not only do family gatherings highlight the new gap or gaps caused by those absent, but the jollity of others can jar painfully. The festivities exposed our raw emotions but it also gave us a chance to be together. Cynthia

[6] Duncan, Alice, *Alice Duncan*, White Bridge Press, Oxford, 2006

was supported by three of her children and their families in Yorkshire. Ronald and I joined Felicity, Alex, Max and Ben in Kidlington. Instead of the usual gaudy Christmas decorations, Felicity had filled the house with flowers and there were lots of photographs by Alice on the walls.

Into the New Year, life went on as it always must. Park Farm was put on the market in the early summer of 2005; Cynthia prepared to move south to her London flat and our family's long Yorkshire chapter came to an end.

And then came my third bolt from the blue.

Part Three
My Cancer

8

Suspicion and Diagnosis

THE FIELDS WERE white with narcissi, the woods pink with
cyclamen. Ronald and I were on our annual walking holiday
with six friends, this time in the Cévennes. In stamina we ranged
from a serious 20-mile walker to the two who had to follow by
car after just a short stroll on the flat. Julia Gregson and I were
somewhere in the middle of this group and our talk was often as
absorbing as the walk. It was a clear sunny day with the
mountains stretching as far as we could see. Our lives felt happy
and secure. We had no qualms about looking to the future.

Both our husbands were in their mid-seventies. Julia is 17
years younger than Richard; I am 13 years younger than
Ronald. Julia and I were both healthy and relatively vigorous. It
was reasonable to expect that we would outlive our husbands,
probably by many years. We discussed the travels we might then
do together, expeditions already unattractive to our partners.
Some, like riding across Mongolia, would never have appealed
to mine. Julia and I were soon quite carried away in the planning of these jaunts.

Six weeks later, in June 2005, this merry widowhood was in
jeopardy.

*

Ronald is very keen on marinades. He will often put great thought and effort into the ingredients, which usually include a wide selection of herbs from the garden. Other times he will just use a jar of exotic oriental sauce from the supermarket. This Thursday evening it was a quick fix with chicken portions in one of those lurid concoctions.

When my dawn visit to the lavatory revealed strangely coloured urine I immediately blamed his oriental sauce. I casually enquired whether he had had the same experience. He said no, which just made me think that his metabolism was slower or different from mine.

I thought little more of it until, when lunching with friends in Ludlow a few hours later, I was surprised to find myself asking for only a small helping of the fish pie. Barbara is the best fish-pie maker I know. By the evening I was definitely feeling queasy; Ronald remained disconcertingly healthy and hungry. By then I had started questioning what, other than the oriental sauce, could be blamed.

That night I had a carefree sleep but the next morning I knew that I had obstructive jaundice. Not only was my urine becoming an increasingly dark brown, my faeces were the classic 'clay colour' that I remembered from my medical school textbook. Ronald confirmed that the 'whites' of my eyes were a faint yellow.

I knew only too well the most likely cause of obstructive jaundice in a 63-year-old woman who had not been outside Europe in the last six months: cancer of the pancreas. The other common, and much less worrying causes, were difficult to entertain. I had felt well so it was unlikely to be any kind of infectious hepatitis. I had always had an iron constitution and hardly knew what indigestion was. A gallstone blocking my bile duct would be very surprising, although by far the most cheerful diagnosis. . . and the one that I chose to focus on in my more optimistic moments or when talking to friends. However a visit to my dusty and very heavy tome on internal medicine revealed a disappointingly short list of rival diagnoses to pancreatic cancer – most of them extremely rare.

I am a great planner. Many of my plans never materialise but I enjoy making them. Indeed it seems I am unable not to plan. Within days of my brief and only pregnancy, I had a daughter on her way to university. Friends often ask us how a holiday has gone when it had actually never got past the planning stage. We had given such thought and talk to it that they naturally assumed it must have taken place.

Thus once pancreatic cancer was on my mind I had leapt ahead planning my way through the most likely scenarios, which were mostly gloomy. I was quite interested in my reaction to this diagnosis. It was not fear or anger. The main one was of disappointment, profound disappointment.

Disappointment that I might not have long to savour this new phase of life that Ronald and I were particularly enjoying. Ronald had recovered far beyond our hopes. We loved our new timber-built home, the garden was flourishing, the fruit and vegetables prolific. We both had enough work to stimulate us and interesting overseas travels as a result. Our work was flexible and neither of us felt stressed by it. We now had much more time for family and friends.

I also felt miffed that I should have put such effort, pain and money into avoiding breast and ovarian cancer only to be hit by another one. I later came to accept this more philosophically; there were, in fact, a number of advantages. Not least, I may well have enjoyed extra years of health by postponing the onset of what would probably have been a much earlier cancer in an ovary or breast.

Finally, I worried about the effect my ill health would have on others. My thoughts turned to Ronald first. Not only was he considerably older and therefore could reasonably have expected me to be there to care for him in the future, but through his own long struggle with cancer I had taken on various, if limited, caring roles. I had been doing most of the driving and the nearest – and infrequent – bus was a very steep hill away.

I also worried about my two nieces, Lizzie and Catherine, now aged 20 and 17. I had never played a parental role in their lives but we were very close and my illness would be bound to bring back sad memories of their own mother's illness and death.

And then there was my sister, Felicity, who had had so much illness and loss to cope with during the last few years. Not only would she be worried for me, but she would have to take over the time-consuming and emotionally draining task of selling our family home in Yorkshire.

On the other hand, if this blow had to fall, I felt intensely relieved by the timing. Few people, other than Ronald, would be inconvenienced. I no longer had any administrative duties at work and therefore no responsibility for the lives of those with whom I worked. I had given up my clinical work some years before so there were no patients to worry about and my days of organising conferences were thankfully over.

Suspicion and Diagnosis

Had I been ill during my father's lifetime, he would have been greatly distressed. I should have been upset myself not to be able to nurse him through his terminal illness and I would have been deprived of the very precious time we had together.

I had at this point no definite diagnosis and it was of course possible that I was overstating the danger. I am conscious, perhaps not sufficiently, that I tend to exaggerate. Rarely do I underplay a story. Having told Ronald and one or two close friends of my fear, I suddenly worried that I was being melo-dramatic and ridiculously began to dread the humiliation of being told that a little benign polyp or stricture was the cause of my trouble.

My emotions were absurdly confused. Good news would be professionally humiliating. Bad news would be bad, perhaps very bad indeed.

Nevertheless, much of the time I tried to convince myself that my robust health, lack of weight loss – indeed, continuing struggle to avoid the 11-stone mark – meant that nothing serious could be afoot. I still intended to go to a housewarming party that evening to which we had been greatly looking forward. By midday it was clear that this was not to be. I would be a dismal guest and certainly wouldn't feel like eating anything.

We have been unusually blessed with our neighbours, the Griffiths; who have become close friends over the years. Our five-acre patch of a high hillside adjoins their 12 acres and we offer shared grazing for a local farmer's sheep. During May Sarah and I share the flower duties for our church. At the weekend we take it in turns to collect the Sunday papers. On this Sunday Sarah delivered our paper and was, I expect, as surprised as I was, when I found myself choking with tears as I anxiously asked if her husband, our GP, would be taking the surgery in the village the next morning.

No one could ask for a better family doctor. Richard immediately rang me and I was seen at 8.30 on the Monday morning. By 11.30 I was having an ultrasound scan in the private hospital in Hereford, 10 miles away.

I seem to be quite good at accepting bad news and even pain. I am hopeless at coping with uncertainty. My years of struggling with infertility had more than demonstrated this to me. I was therefore willing to pay quite a lot to avoid the days, even weeks, of inevitable delay that there would have been had I gone with the National Health Service.

The scan confirmed the obstruction to the bile duct but gave no indication as to what was causing it. I then met the surgeon in Hereford, who said that the next stage was to have a look at my bile duct through a telescope that he would insert via my stomach and duodenum, the piece of gut that links the stomach to the main coils of the small intestine.

He hoped to be able to put a stent into my bile duct at the same time in order to clear the obstruction and therefore my jaundice. I was relieved to hear this. By now I was quite definitely yellow and, of much more concern, feeling queasy and lethargic with no appetite at all. The loss of appetite was the least of the worries. Indeed it gave me ironic pleasure to see the pounds I had been struggling and failing to lose over many years slip away in 10 days.

I was sent a letter with an appointment for the next week for the procedure, an ERCP. When I gently, if condescendingly, suggested they might spell this out for non-medical clients –

without admitting that I hadn't a clue what it meant myself – the secretary replied 'Do you feel that it would help people if we wrote endoscopic retrograde cholangio-pancreatography?' I had to admit that it probably wouldn't.

This further examination confirmed that what was blocking the bile duct was a tumour in the pancreas. It was not possible at that stage to know whether this was a primary tumour starting in the pancreas, or a secondary cancer that had spread from some other part of my body. Unfortunately the tumour had distorted the bile duct so the stent could not be inserted to relieve the obstruction and therefore stop the jaundice. My delight in weight loss was now seriously qualified by my increasing nausea and lethargy.

A CT or computerised tomography scan was the next step and was arranged for three days' time. This showed more detail and was somewhat reassuring in that it suggested that the tumour had not spread outside the pancreas and was therefore more likely to be fully removable.

Ronald and I discussed the situation with the surgeon, who was very straight with us from the start. He described what sounded like a daunting operation involving the removal of much of my pancreas, my gall bladder and a chunk of bowel, the duodenum. Although he told us he had done this operation himself he was firm in his advice that we should go to a specialist centre where not just the surgeons but all the support staff were involved with such operations on a daily basis. In the Liver Unit in the Birmingham University Hospital four surgeons spent most of their time on surgery involving the liver and pancreas.

Up until now it was only family and those friends who happened to be in touch with us over that fortnight who knew that I was unwell. Felicity had been as concerned as I would have expected. She, like the rest of the family, was shocked by the turn of events. They had never known me ill. She wrote to a friend in New York.

Frankly, when it happened I could not believe it.

Libby is the one who never gets ill. She is the one we turn to and rely on and who looks after all of us. She is also the sensible one. When Bunny had ovarian cancer Libby had her ovaries removed; when I had breast cancer she had her breasts removed. Cancer of the pancreas could be connected with that same wretched gene.

It has certainly jolted me out of my own self-absorption.

As I was clearly going to be out of action for some time Ronald and I discussed what we would now say and to whom. We agreed that we wanted to be open from the start both about facts and also about our feelings and fears. So I wrote to my close friends and made it clear that they could share the news with anyone who might be interested.

Who to send it to was a bit problematic – it seemed an imposition to bore or burden those who didn't know us well, but we didn't want anyone to feel left out. We probably erred in both directions. Anyway this is the letter I sent by email or post:

My very dear friends

Considering my usual buoyant health, I am afraid this letter may come as a shock to some of you. For others it is just a further instalment on a problem that started out of the blue two weeks ago. I became jaundiced and a blocked bile duct was found to be the cause. Yesterday it was confirmed that this blockage was due to a tumour in my pancreas. With our family experiences, this is not a shock but it is a very big disappointment.

However the good news is that it looks as if it has been caught early and there is no reason why it shouldn't be completely removed. It will be quite a big operation and I hope to go into hospital within two weeks.

I (briefly) wondered whether to tell you but realised that I had no choice as Ronald and I will badly need your loving support over the next few weeks. I also wanted you to realise just how much your friendship means to me. Some of you are friends from my earliest childhood, others are new friends, but I treasure you all and am only sorry to have to burden you yet again when many of you gave so much support through our family sadnesses last year. Nurse Higgins is caring, loving and calm but will value your support as much as I will. As well as Ronald, I am of course worried about Lizzie and Catherine, Bunny's children, and indeed about Felicity. I am sure that those of you who know them well will be there for them too. (Catherine is just off to Peru for six weeks so will be out of touch for a bit.)

I am only writing to a small group of very close friends but if you feel there are other people who might like to know please feel free to tell them.

I may well be off email when in hospital but messages will always reach me via Ronald.

Please don't feel that any action on your part is needed. Your caring thoughts are all we need.

With very much love to you all

Libby

To my godchildren, by then all adults, I sent an amended version.

Dear Christopher, David, Emily, Sam, Vicki, Fiona, Tanya, Caroline, Hetty, Amanda, Emily, Katie and Thomas (in chronological order!)

I know that some of you have already heard of the unwelcome happening in my life: that this week, after only a few days of illness, I have been found to have a tumour of the pancreas. Fortunately this has been caught early and should be completely removable but will need some quite major surgery within the next two weeks or so. Nurse Higgins is showing previously untested talents and I feel very well cared for and expect to be back in full action by the end of the year.

However this shock has made me realise just how much I treasure my friends and not least my godchildren. Although I have not always been as attentive as I should have liked, I have followed all your doings with such interest – and really appreciate how every one of you has kept in touch with me. I have so many happy memories of times together, none greater than the ones from the 'camps' in Rosedale. I now have 16 grand-godchildren and I love to hear of their doings too.

Please don't feel that you need take any action in response to this letter. Your caring thoughts are all I need. However, the thing that would give me the greatest pleasure is a recent photograph of you and/or children. My last photo of some of you was either at the camp in Rosedale or at your weddings!

With very much love to you all

Libby

We have never regretted this decision to be open. Some of our friends may well have felt they were told more than they wanted to know, and certainly in greater detail. But for us the continuing support and encouragement of our friends is what kept us going in lower moments.

We now had to make a decision between treatment in Birmingham, 75 miles from home, or in London which was 150 miles away. This would not only be for the two weeks or so of the operation but the probable follow-up treatment of at least six months. An added factor in the equation was Ronald's restricted driving range due to his leg problem; but at least that could get us both to our nearest railway station, Hereford.

London was the natural choice. I had worked there for many years and I still had an honorary appointment at Hammersmith Hospital. We had many friends in London. We both had plenty to do there. We didn't know Birmingham well. Furthermore Birmingham was where Bunny's family lived and where she herself had lived and died. Rob and the children had spent several years visiting the Cancer Unit there. I hated the idea of unnecessarily kindling sad memories for them.

On the other hand the inevitable lack of personal communication between a distant London specialist and my family doctor during my infertility treatment and, much more recently, after my mastectomy, had caused real problems. In the case of my mastectomy I believed it had contributed to the poor outcome.

We soon decided that the obvious advantages of London were outweighed by the excellent relationship between the specialist in Hereford and the Birmingham team in the same NHS region. He knew all the surgeons well, clearly had a high regard for them and had frequently shared patients. He was also a friend as well as a colleague of my GP. I felt I could trust them all to keep in close touch and this has proved true.

Having made that decision, we got in touch with the hospital in Birmingham, the results of all my investigations were sent over and an outpatient appointment was made for the following week with a view to being put on the waiting list for surgery. By now I was desperate to get the operation over. This was partly because I was feeling horrid but even more because of my impatience to know the nature and spread of the tumour, and therefore the probable long-term outlook.

Yet again, I felt blessed by the timing of this otherwise unwelcome happening. Our dear friends Patrick and Marilyn Pietroni had that very week moved from France to Shropshire, only an hour away from Birmingham. Patrick, who had supported us through so many stresses in the past, immediately abandoned the unpacking to spend the day with me in the Birmingham outpatient clinic.

On a hot July morning Patrick and I sat ourselves down in the Birmingham hospital's pokey and crowded Liver Clinic. Expecting a long wait, he went off to survey the large choice of leaflets displayed on the counter. He returned with two copies of 'Surgery for Pancreatic Cancer – Patient Information Booklet' – all 16 pages of it. We read intently and in silence for five minutes – then found ourselves incongruously laughing, crying being the only alternative. The candour of the writing could only be admired.

The cure rate for pancreatic cancer is one in five patients, who have had their cancer resected successfully. The remaining four will have the cancer back within about two years.

Then followed clear descriptions and diagrams of the three possible operations which were described as 'major surgery' or 'very major surgery'. All were likely to lead to digestion problems, and one of them to diabetes and a susceptibility to infection. 'Getting over this type of surgery is hard work', as the brochure put it, seemed something of an understatement. Further on the booklet gave a very full description of what would happen and why, after the operation and during the rest of the stay in hospital.

Then followed a list of possible post-operative complications such as bleeding, leaking and infection, all of which seemed to occur in a disconcertingly high proportion of candidates. The section ended with the warning that despite the recent reduction in complications in specialist centres '5–9 per cent of people die directly as a result of complications after their operation'.

We were then told that 'in about four cases out of 10, it is not possible to remove the cancer, even though your specialist thought resection was possible.' The booklet ended with several pages on what could be done for those whose tumour could not be removed.

Armed with this daunting knowledge we were ushered into the presence of the Liver Surgeon, Mr Darius Mirza.

Throughout the booklet there had been encouraging phrases: 'Do ask as many questions as you need to', 'Don't worry if you think of more questions later, just speak to your nurses', 'The specialist nurse is always available for questions and her contact details are. . . '.

Too often I have heard patients say that, when it came to it, the doctor gave them no real chance to ask questions. Here, the opposite was true. I almost felt I would disappoint Mr Mirza if I didn't think up some more. Whenever he paused for breath, he would say, 'Any questions?'

I was immediately reassured. I knew that I was in the right hands and that I was happy to follow his advice. Actually there were few decisions to make. The tumour should be, and probably could be, removed. I wanted it out as soon as possible. I had been told that the waiting list for this particular surgery was likely to be at least two or three weeks. And even then I must be prepared for a last-minute postponement to allow for an urgent, inevitably unpredictable, liver transplant.

But again I was in luck. Because the operating theatres were to have been closed for refurbishing the following week, no operations had been booked. Unexpectedly the contractors had postponed their work. The operating list was a blank sheet. Could I possibly come into hospital on Sunday, which was two days later, for surgery on Monday? I leapt at the opportunity. My only hesitation was Ronald's birthday on the Sunday; a day of us sitting in the hospital would hardly be the celebration of choice. I explained this dilemma.

My wonderfully accommodating surgeon immediately suggested that I should instead spend that very day going through all the necessary admission routine of examination, blood tests, X-rays and ECGs. Then I could come in as late as I liked on Sunday evening, preferably, he added, by midnight!

So Patrick and I had a surprisingly uplifting day, something of a treasure hunt, as we searched out the requisite departments through the maze of corridors and lifts, helped by the cheerful colour coding which livened up what would otherwise be a very gloomy thirties building. At each reception desk we were expected and welcomed and one radiographer even knew it was to be my husband's birthday. It is perhaps surprising quite how much these personal touches mean at a sensitive time. I am sure they had a lasting effect on my feelings about Birmingham health care.

A delightful medical student on a secondment from France took my admission details and gave me the routine admission examination. Memories of my own medical student days and the excitement of having one's first patient surged back. (Actually mine, back in the sixties, was a bit of a problem. I could never catch her awake and was much too nervous to wake her – I would like to think this was compassion on my part but that would not be true.) Sadly this was the first and last medical student I was to meet in the next six months.

The formalities fulfilled, the tasks completed, I returned home that Friday evening feeling profoundly thankful that I had only three days to wait. Any fear I had of the surgeon's knife was submerged by impatience to learn what it would reveal.

9

Waiting for Surgery

IN THE THREE weeks from the appearance of my first symptoms to my admission to hospital, life and the necessary adjustments to it continued.

First, the house needed to be prepared for my convalescence. This could have caused friction between Ronald and me. I assume all marriages have their tensions, MTs as we call them. Wise friends could no doubt have told us long ago that some of ours would never be resolved. Yet we each determinedly persevere with our own views. We have a room, described by the architect as a 'day room', which has been the cause of one of our most enduring and vigorous disagreements. This room is an attractive, oak-timbered conservatory leading directly from our bedroom into the garden.

Ronald considers it a perfect greenhouse where tender seedlings can have ready access to the 24-hour nurturing of their often pyjama-clad master. Whereas for me the idea of being able to wake early and tiptoe out to a chaise longue from where I can look out at the Black Mountains is equally attractive.

As Ronald had spent a great deal more time gardening than

146

I ever had lying on a chaise longue, he had, not surprisingly, won this particular battle of wills from the beginning. By the time of my illness there was no question of space for such a grand piece of furniture. To find a place among the pots and seedboxes for so much as the smallest upright chair would have been a challenge.

It therefore took careful planning of arguments and choice of moment, to lodge my request. I finally chose a mutually sleepless period at around three in the morning. I pointed out that in the next few months I was likely to have far more time for lying on a chaise longue and that he, in his new caring role, far less time for propagating plants. Furthermore, as the downstairs of our house is largely open plan, the conservatory was the only room, other than our bedroom, in which I would be able to see my visitors with any privacy. Might there now be a possible case for a change in its function?

The very idea of this transformation had a soporific effect on Ronald. Within minutes my sleepless longings were accompanied by peaceful snoring from the body by my side. I dared hope no more.

It was therefore a complete surprise when two exhausted but triumphant men appeared at my bedside the next afternoon: Ronald, of course, and our one-day-a-week Kikuyun Kenyan gardener, Guama. Guama is as strong as he is cheerful; the perfect companion for a physically and emotionally challenging task. In four hours, the greenhouse had become a conservatory. The chaise longue and a table with a telephone upon it had replaced the seed trays. There were even two chairs for visitors and a decorative screen hid the last vestiges of gardening equipment. No greater love could a husband have shown. The sacrifice for him was great and much appreciated; this room was to become my haven for many months.

When, the following day, Frances Hancock came to celebrate Holy Communion with Ronald and me it seemed fitting that the conservatory should be our chapel, a christening for its new life. Frances arrived in the village next to ours in Herefordshire just before Bunny died. She had helped me then, and again when my father died. Like Bunny, Frances had been one of the first women to be ordained as a priest. In her early sixties she had been a welcome addition to our parish clergy as well as being the bishop's adviser on women in ministry in the diocese. Although I had not known her well I had always admired the dignity of this tall, white-haired woman and nearly always went home with a helpful message from her sermons. Her quiet composure and self-containment concealed warmth, fun and humour, which I was to discover over the coming year.

We have another ongoing MT: the television. Ronald is a much keener television watcher than I am. Not only is he interested in every detail of every cricket, football, rugby and tennis match but he is an avid collector of garden tips and recipes. Nor is any day complete without several instalments of the news. As reading a novel is a relaxation for me, so is watching television for him.

When we built our house we spent large sums on having a beautifully designed 'built in' covered television/video/CD/bookcase in our bedroom. This worked well until a misguided friend introduced Ronald to plasma television screens and the possibility of turning one's bedroom effectively into a cinema. The slot for the television in our covered unit, now being far too small for its original purpose, was duly filled with books. The plasma screen then replaced several large attractive pictures higher on the wall.

These pictures had been carefully positioned to give maximum pleasure to anyone as they entered the room. Now, with some leftover curtain material, I rather lamely made a cover for the new appendage hoping people might be deceived into thinking it was another window.

Until now I had of course been under no obligation to watch the television. For the following few weeks I was unlikely to be able to escape. But ever sensitive to my needs, Ronald discovered some splendid earphones that he could attach to the television so at least there was no sound. A huge improvement, but I still found the flickering screen a distraction from reading. We are still working on the ideal pulley system which could lower a curtain around me so that I can remain by his side in bed with neither auditory nor visual distraction.

Next our diaries had to be adjusted. June and July are busy months at Quercwm. The garden is at its most fruitful and floriferous. Weeding and soft fruit picking are essential daily activities. It is also the time when we tend to most welcome visitors. Weekends are planned well ahead.

That year Lizzie, my 20-year-old photography student niece, was needing to boost her funds so we had arranged that she should come and help with the fruit picking, cooking and entertaining for two weekends running. Providentially these turned out to be the very two weekends that I was lying in waiting for surgery. She was a godsend. She provided domestic help to Ronald and comfort to me.

So the first weekend went ahead as arranged. It had been carefully planned as Lalage Neal, a psychotherapist who had given me so much help and guidance in my own counselling of bereaved families in London, was coming. This was her first visit since the death of her husband, John Percival, from cancer only six months earlier. Although Ronald and I did not know John well, we shared some close friends and it was they who were joining us for Sunday lunch. I was determined that nothing should prevent this.

The third visitor that weekend was Jean Curtis Raleigh. Jean is a friend and psychiatrist who had given wise and loving support to us all through Alice's illness. In another role, as a mother of twin boys, she had been involved with the Multiple Births Foundation since its inception and was now one of its trustees. Coincidentally Lalage had worked with Jean during her training days and this was a happy reunion for them. Jean, Lalage and Lizzie proved a perfect trio, getting to know each other far better without my presence than they might otherwise have done. Since then Lizzie and Lalage's daughter Nell, also an art student, have become friends.

Meanwhile, I lay in bed listening to laughter and snatches of nostalgic reminiscences. After the Sunday lunch one friend after another popped in to see me. It was lovely to know they would be with me on this journey whatever its destination.

The second weekend was to have been our annual summer garden lunch, when 60 or so friends should have been gathering on the lawn. This was cancelled, partly because I would not have been able to help with the considerable work involved, but also because my still uncertain diagnosis might have caused some awkwardness. During this time friends were tending to polarise into the pessimist and optimist groups. Casual mingling over summer pudding and white wine might have been less easy than usual.

The only visitors, other than Lizzie, who were not cancelled for this second weekend were Ronald's brother and his wife, Peter and Geraldine. No summer party ever takes place without them. They have the two vital qualities that Ronald and I are short of and often lose entirely on the morning of such parties: calmness and efficiency. Peter does every last-minute odd job, such as organising the car park and putting up signs for the loo. During the party he mans the bar while Geraldine puts together the final food titivations and keeps the kitchen in order. They both then quietly remind us of everything that we have forgotten.

Now Peter and Geraldine were equally welcome for a more peaceful weekend which turned into the gathering of the family. Felicity with her usual generosity cancelled everything and brought her younger son Ben down from Oxford, picking up our niece Catherine from the Birmingham train in Hereford.

The fourth of the younger generation, Max, Ben's older brother, had telephoned and we spoke for a long time together. I was profoundly touched by the attentiveness and caring of all four of my nephews and nieces. This weekend was particularly important to me as three of them were just about to set off on their travels. Catherine was going to Peru for six weeks, Lizzie for a month in New York and Ben was spending a month in Wyoming. I was so glad that they should see me now looking okay. Indeed they thought that the 'suntan' suited me well. By the time they returned I expected to be fit again. And should I not be there on their return, they would, I hoped, have happy memories of our weekend together.

During that weekend I had good conversations in the conservatory with each of my young visitors. Any idea that they should be shielded from yet another family setback was ridiculous. They were all too generous. They would be offended by such protection. I treasure a letter from Catherine before she went abroad in which she wrote: 'I hope you will always tell me everything, otherwise I shall imagine the worst.' It was a permission, indeed a request, for which I was deeply grateful. I know that I would not have been as brave and open with my aunts when I was 17.

They have all four shown extraordinary sensitivity and resilience to the losses and worries that they have had to face in their short lives. Nor have any of them tried to avoid them. At no time was this better exemplified than Lizzie's remark in our kitchen that weekend. They were gathered there with Felicity and someone commented that it seemed hard that our family should have so many afflictions. To which Lizzie responded 'Yes, but just look how it brings us all together.' She is right. With our diverse lives and personalities, I am quite sure that we are closer as a family than we would have been had we had these same privileged lives but without the pains.

I have talked to people with cancer and read of many more. Reactions seem to vary so widely. From shock, denial, defeat and fear to anger, guilt and failure. All uncomfortable to live with and emotions that I, largely and thankfully, didn't suffer from.

For a number of reasons I was lucky. I had had something of a trial run. I had faced and coped reasonably well with a far greater loss than death in my sixties, that of childlessness in my thirties. Had I been offered the choice of which to be spared, I would have had no doubts, even now. In the same way I understand better now how Felicity seemed to treat her cancer so lightly. An 18-year-old daughter with a severe mental illness was an incomparably greater worry than her own potentially life-threatening illness.

Had I had a heart attack or some other grave illness, I should certainly have been shocked but cancer, no. I had lived for so many years in its shadow that for it finally to emerge was not a surprise but, as I have already said, just a big disappointment. There was little risk of denial. I was much too interested in my cancer and how it affected me.

I never suffered from anger and the 'why me?' syndrome. I had been saying a different 'why me?' for many years. Why, when carrying the same cancer gene as my two younger sisters was it me that had been spared for so long? If anything, I should have been the most vulnerable. Breastfeeding is known to reduce the risk of some forms of breast cancer. I had had no children to breastfeed. My sisters had breastfed five children between them. And unlike Felicity and Bunny, I had never taken the contraceptive pill which is known to reduce the risks of ovarian cancer. Instead I had had various hormones to stimulate my ovaries during my treatment for infertility, a factor known to increase the chances of developing a malignant tumour.

Together with 'why me?' may come 'it's not fair'. This thought, should it have arisen, I would have instantly dismissed as irrelevant. I had learnt long ago, through many wonderful patients, that life is not fair and that there is absolutely no correlation between physical suffering and either virtue or vice.

In fact I tended more to say 'why not me?' On the lifeboat principle, where the least useful member is chosen to go overboard to allow others to survive, I had no difficulty in seeing that I should be the one chosen. I had no children who would be bereft. My main work in life was completed. I had wonderful support from my husband, family and friends.

Perhaps most important of all, I might be able to put the experience to good use. Few people could have been better prepared. I had medical training behind me, even if my knowledge of pancreatic cancer was very rusty indeed, and certainly outdated. But at least it gave me a curiosity about the whole experience and this helped to protect me through my treatment over the next year. Whenever things got horrid, I could usually detach myself and think of it as an interesting 'other side of the fence' experience.

And I am sure that the idea of my own death was less bewildering for me than for many people. Not only had I worked with bereaved families, I had also had the privilege of accompanying two people who had no fear of death, my sister and my father, through the last weeks of their lives. This had undoubtedly helped to remove any fear that death might have held for me.

Guilt was never a problem. Although there is no certainty that pancreatic cancer is related to our family's BRCA1 cancer gene, I couldn't help feeling that it was likely. That assumption may well, however illogically, have protected me from any feelings of guilt that this cancer was of my own doing. Of course I know that environmental influences, including diet, can influence the appearance of a cancer even when it is primarily determined by one's genes. For instance, it is not yet understood why some people who carry the BRCA1 cancer gene survive into old age with no sign of cancer while the majority show it much earlier in life.

Others might say I should not have relieved myself of guilt

so easily. Especially in view of my life-long addiction to coffee. The section on pancreatic cancer in my medical tome says that 'Excessive caffeine consumption has also been implicated'. I understand that more recent research has not confirmed an association. And anyway it had never occurred to me that my pancreas was at risk. Ovaries and breasts, yes, but my pancreas I had never even thought about. Nevertheless I have always known that my caffeine consumption was unwisely high. Sporadic efforts to reduce or even eliminate it have been pathetically unsuccessful. I am ashamed of this, especially when I am intolerant of those who continue to smoke cigarettes.

I was also spared uninvited comments from other people as to why I might have been chosen as a cancer victim. Other friends with cancer have told me that they really resented suggestions such as 'you've always had such stressful jobs, it's not surprising' or even 'maybe you have been suppressing your anger'. The family cancer gene was all too evident in my case.

Perhaps, if I am honest, my main negative reaction may have been that of too easy acceptance, a form of defeat. I felt tired in spirit, perhaps not helped by the jaundice. I had tried so hard to avoid cancer. Now it was here, how hard could I go on trying? Was it time just to be grateful for all I had had? It was perhaps greedy to ask for more.

Now, one year later it is not difficult to write about these feelings with some dispassion. At the time, of course, they were much more confused and there were a lot of tears and fears and suspense. And little things loomed absurdly large. I spent more time worrying about my shame at the thought of Ronald seeing and trying to sort the chaos in my study than worrying about the death that would give him this predicament.

I did try to get a bit organised. I updated my will. I discussed funeral arrangements, my hymns, who might take the service, who would say a few words, those sort of preparations which would hopefully take the pressure off Ronald. We had always talked of being cremated. It seemed tidier and more economical in space. But a recent article showing the energy consumed by crematoria as well as our increasing awareness of the dangers of pollution and global warming has given us pause. The decision, currently at least, is to be buried in a biodegradable coffin. Cardboard, pine, bamboo or willow seem to be the options. Photographs of willow ones looked beautiful but seemed extravagant for an article viewed for such a short time. I decided on bamboo. Several websites give instructions on do-it-yourself coffins. I haven't told Ronald this. He may be tempted to use our newly planted bamboo copse.

Practical problems arose. Our lovely church in Vowchurch is small. My family is large and we have a wide circle of friends, most of whom still have busy lives, many in London or Yorkshire. Short notice would be difficult for their diaries, travel would be awkward and especially, without being too conceited, if there wouldn't be a seat for them once they arrived. Most of all, the contingency plans for an invasion from London and Yorkshire would be daunting for Ronald.

Far better it seemed would be to have a funeral in Vowchurch just for family and local friends. Later, there could be a thanksgiving service for other friends and colleagues in London. I liked to think that this would also be a happy reunion for Multiple Birth Foundation friends, for some of the volunteer parents who had contributed so much and become such good friends over the years. Just as we had a guard of honour of 25 pairs of young twins at our wedding, perhaps their parents would cheer me on to my next journey.

These were my plans if I failed to return from hospital or died soon after. Clearly such elaborate ideas would become irrelevant in a few years. My now active friends would be fewer in number and less able to travel. Few would remember my many happy years with multiple birth families. The pew space in Vowchurch would then be more than adequate for my send off.

During these brief weeks I was deeply touched by the surge of loving concern and offers of help from neighbours and friends. All wanted to support. Most got it right. A few got it wrong, usually the over cheerful. Comments such as '*you* are bound to be fine' or 'you are strong, and it's mind over matter' were irritating. Why was I any more likely than anyone else to be among the small group who survive pancreatic cancer? Yes I would of course try to be one of the lucky few but it would surely have been arrogant to assume I had any more right to that privileged position than anyone else

Among my many wonderful friends, there was inevitably something very special about the mutual support of a fellow traveller, not that I would have wished it on anyone, let alone a very close friend. Sue Norrington lives in the next valley and her arrival in this part of Herefordshire has brought pleasure to us all and music to that valley, with the three concerts she arranges every year in aid of the beautiful 14th-century church of Craswall.

For several months Sue had felt unusually tired and generally unwell and had been having various investigations to try to find out the cause. I had been keeping in close, if ineffectual, touch. When it was discovered that she had a cancer of the bowel, I was as shocked and upset as her many other friends. She was to have an operation in London and said she would come to supper a day or two before.

Ronald and I prepared to give what support we could, never guessing that by the time we met I too would be waiting for abdominal surgery. I can still see the scene on that summer evening on our terrace, neither of us able to eat much, with indescribable beauty around us, neither of us knowing what the future held and whether we would be here again this time next year.

Although I have had periods in my life when prayer was part of my daily regime, these periods have been relatively infrequent and short-lived. Mostly prayer has been when with others in church or on my own during times of crisis, sadness and sometimes, not often enough, in times of wonder and happiness. I would have expected that prayer would be important to me now. It wasn't. Somehow I found little comfort in praying myself but I did get huge comfort from knowing how many generous friends were holding me in their prayers. I was touched too by the thought that I was being remembered for many weeks at the Sunday service in my own village church.

When I did manage to pray it was never for a cure, but for the strength and serenity to accept what was to be.

> O God, grant me the serenity to accept the things I cannot change,
> Courage to change the things I can,
> And wisdom to know the difference.
>
> Reinhold Niebuhr

IO

Taken by Surprise

I HAVE BEEN writing the last two chapters during the second half of June and early July 2006, the same weeks in which, the year before, I had changed from being someone in perfect health to one with a life-threatening disease.

Each day over these three weeks has, in a sense, been an anniversary. Each of these anniversaries I remember with the detail and clarity of only the most memorable celebrations or catastrophes in the rest of my life. As I have written about it, I have lived each day again. I believe I have not only been telling the story but remembering it as it was.

I am not doubting the accuracy of my memory or the honesty of my reporting, but I am suddenly amazed by my feelings at that time. How could I have been so relatively calm then, when today I feel shattered and Ronald has been mopping up the tears?

On the one hand much is unchanged. I am glad to report that I am still allowed to enjoy the chaise longue in the conservatory. The garden, as is its wont in early July, is again overwhelming us with its bounty. The soft-fruit crop is now upon us and I am again pointing out to Ronald that we still have half of last year's crop in the freezer and are rapidly running out of friends in need of blackcurrant jelly. Jean Curtis Raleigh has come again for her annual concert visit.

On the other hand everything this morning changed. I was suddenly hit by the terrifying fragility of this wondrous life. As I sat listening to the dawn chorus my impersonal computer was coldly telling me that the chance of my continuing to enjoy this life was small. I had logged on to the Internet to research this chapter and my findings were grim. It was a shock to my system. There have been periods when my life was perhaps more exciting, more stimulating, in some ways more obviously rewarding than it is now. But it has never been happier. The thought that it might be cut short is hard to face. Perhaps there is no point in dwelling on it. But sometimes I can't stop myself.

How can I explain the suddenness and depth of this shock? Here was I, an NHS consultant who had seen serious or fatal cancers develop in several members of my family. I'd read all those depressingly frank documents at the Liver Unit and talked it all through with knowledgeable medical colleagues as well as my own surgeons and physicians. I should have been fully prepared to face all the facts, swallow hard and recognise how gloomy the statistics on survival would read. I was not prepared.

Most people will know someone, even a relative or close friend, with breast cancer. Far fewer will know someone with pancreatic cancer, which is hardly surprising. While the breast comes top of the cancer league with 23 per cent of all cancers in women, the pancreas is way down at eleventh with a score of only 3 per cent. Around 41,700 women are diagnosed with breast cancer each year compared to about 3,500 women with pancreatic cancer. The risk of being diagnosed with pancreatic cancer at some point in your life is 1 in 95 for women. For breast cancer it is 1 in 9 and for ovarian cancer 1 in 48.

In addition to this low incidence, you are much less likely to bump into a 'walking wounded' with pancreatic cancer and even less likely to meet a cured person. The victims rarely last long whereas now nearly 80 per cent of breast cancer sufferers survive for over five years after their initial diagnosis.

It is not difficult to find websites on every sort of cancer. You are spoilt for choice. I chose that of Cancer Research UK and went straight to the section on cancer of the pancreas. I went to the subsection marked 'for professionals'. Before entering this, patients are advised to redirect themselves to a more suitable location. Presumably one where the pill has a sugar coating.

The facts were clear and stark. I was told that 'the proportion of people surviving pancreatic cancer is very low, and the length of time between diagnosis and death is typically short, at usually less than six months. The most recent data for patients diagnosed in England and Wales show that around 13 per cent of people with pancreatic cancer survive beyond 12 months after diagnosis and only 2 to 3 per cent beyond five years.

I have always been competitive (and continue to be ferociously so during our daily wake-up table tennis). There are some competitions in my life in which I have come out in the top 20 per cent, perhaps a few in the top 10 per cent, but I can't remember one where I was in the top 2 to 3 per cent. Always a first time, I try to tell myself.

Although there has been some increase over the past 30 years in the number of patients with pancreatic cancer who survive for one year, there has been little, if any, increase in the number who survive for five years. It is a very different picture from breast cancer where the number of people surviving for five years has increased from 52 per cent to 80 per cent over the same period. Not surprisingly, younger patients with pancreatic cancer have a better outlook than older. In my early sixties, I am right in the middle, between the youngest group which is defined as 'under 50' and the oldest of 'over 80'.

The incidence of eight cases of pancreatic cancer per 100,000 women has remained steady over 30 years whereas the incidence in men has fallen from just over 12 cases, to under 10. It is thought that 25 to 30 per cent of cases of pancreatic cancer are related to smoking, which explains the higher but falling rate in men.

Nearly all – about 95 per cent – of pancreatic tumours are of the same type, known as ductal adenocarcinomas, which means that the cells arise from the glands in the pancreas that produce the enzymes to help digestion.

One of the reasons that patients with pancreatic cancer have such a poor outlook is that the patient often doesn't have any warning of it until it has already grown and spread dangerously. Unlike a tumour of the breast or skin, such as a melanoma, there are no visible or palpable signs. The pancreas is deep in the body and much can happen to it without anyone knowing. In the early stages of the cancer's growth, the patient may have no symptoms at all. Later they may feel unwell with symptoms that are not specific enough to direct either patient or doctor to the offending organ.

I was lucky. My tumour was near the bile duct and as soon as the tumour obstructed this I became jaundiced – a very clear and visible sign that something was wrong. And even a signpost to where the trouble lay. This was quite unlike my friend Julia

Trevelyán Oman, who had been unwell for several months before the cause was finally discovered. By then it was too late; the tumour had already spread too widely to be removed.

I must have read all these gloomy statistics last year. I suppose at the time I was so relieved to find that my tumour could be operated on at all that I just ignored the less positive news. Perhaps I just wasn't ready to absorb it. Maybe that was a good thing.

This particular day was the first time for many months that I have felt overwhelmed with anticipatory sorrow. I panicked. If there may be so little time left I must not waste it. Is shutting myself up with my computer the right thing to be doing? Of course the truth is that I am no different from any other person in the world. We may all be living our last days. How can we know? Wasting time thinking about it certainly won't make the remainder of my life any happier, however long or short it turns out to be.

And anyway, Ronald assures me that at the computer is just where I should be. He is not used to having me around during the daytime. He was amazingly tolerant of the interruptions and the flow of demands and visitors during my illness and convalescence. Now it is time for peace, the less I am heard and seen during most of the day, the better.

It is now some time since I wrote this chapter. When I sent it to my friend and literary agent, Carol Heaton, she rang back immediately. She was clearly as concerned for my emotional well-being as about the depressing statistics. Not just because she would regret it if this book didn't get finished; mainly she rang to remind me of her friend in New York who had lived five years after the diagnosis of pancreatic cancer. I felt better for her call.

11

Queen Elizabeth Hospital, Birmingham

SUNDAY 10 JULY 2005 was Ronald's seventy-sixth birthday. It was a big day for me too. We celebrated. It was a beautiful clear sunny morning. Frances gave us Holy Communion on our terrace looking across the sunlit valley at the Black Mountains and surrounded by bird song and rather noisy sheep. She had brought Holy Communion to people in many places, but none, she said, more beautiful. The memory of that service sustained me in the dark hours of the next two weeks and beyond.

But conducting the service cannot have been easy for Frances. Just as I, as a paediatrician, have at times found it especially difficult to care for the very ill child of a close friend so, I imagine, must it be difficult to minister to distressed friends, especially when they have abandoned any effort to hold back their tears.

After lunch we drove up to the Pietronis' home in Shropshire for Ronald's birthday tea. Patrick was to drive us over to the Birmingham hospital in the evening and Ronald would then spend the next few nights with Patrick and Marilyn while I was in hospital.

A surprise awaited us. We were led into the garden. Hidden

among the shrubs was a period piece. Marilyn had created a table that would have won any prize for beauty as well as content. I vividly remembered the impact and atmosphere of this scene but, perhaps partly due to pre-op emotion combined with jaundice, the details were hazy. I asked Marilyn to remind me. This was her reply:

For me too that was a memorable event... We had barely moved in (July 7th) and I had just come home after my knee cartilage op! There were also the terrorist attacks in London...

The tea party was like an oasis of continuity amidst these threats and changes. Sharpened by the fear of losing you, I remember focusing on what would make a light, pretty and enjoyable tea! The old rusty garden furniture was placed in the spot with the best view of the Shropshire Hills and Coalbrookdale power station, and near a birch glade that offered dappled shade in which you placed yourself, dressed in white, behatted and serene! The tables were covered in my mother's ancient white lace cloths, the china was Royal Worcester Howard, white with a bright navy band that matched the deep blue glasses for champagne. Lavender and pink rosebuds on the table, with a little *Alchemilla mollis* as foliage.

Menu: I was playing at an English ethnic tea (having just arrived from France!). Cucumber sandwiches on brown bread, a mousse of salmon trout, crème fraiche and chives, strawberries, meringues and cream. Earl Grey or our favoured dark Yorkshire tea.

Time was running out and we all knew what that meant but had our various treasured memories of the day.

Joining this scene were Danny and Barbara McDowell, close friends ever since my time in York over 30 years ago, who now live only an hour away from us in Ludlow. The visual feast was edifying even if I couldn't actually eat anything. And the birthday boy made up for my deficiencies. Champagne helped us to enjoy the present even more and to look hopefully to the future.

Late that evening Patrick drove Ronald and me to Birmingham. That night I slept reasonably well and I don't remember feeling much anxiety, just relief that something was about to be done. I had hated this limbo period of feeling sick and not knowing fully what was happening inside me. Early on the Monday morning I was collected for theatre.

During five hours in the operating theatre Mr Mirza and his colleagues performed a pylorus-preserving pancreaticoduodenectomy. This is otherwise known as a 'modified Whipple's' operation. This meant that the duodenum was removed together with half my pancreas and my gall bladder. The modification meant that I did not have to lose any of my stomach, for which I was grateful as, not surprisingly, that can seriously add to later difficulties with digestion.

I was lucky too that a good chunk of pancreas could be left behind as I knew that without it I would be bound to develop diabetes – a tedious side effect, to say the least.

The next few days are something of a blur. After the operation I was in the high dependency ward for 48 hours with nine tubes either draining liquids out of various parts of my body or putting anaesthetic or nutrition in. Thanks to my epidural anaesthetic I had little pain and the little I did have was promptly discussed with me and then controlled by a remarkably efficient pain control team.

Now and in the months to come I realised how much easier it had all been for me than for many of my neighbours on the ward. I had had no delay in the diagnosis of my cancer. Some of them had had many weeks, even months of malaise before the reason had been found. Others had had to wait several weeks for their operation and then had it postponed at the last minute to allow for another patient to have a liver transplant that could not be delayed.

But most of all, I was saved from the greatest fear. That of the unknown. I had worked in an intensive care unit. My knowledge was out of date and I didn't understand a lot of the figures on the computer screen but the flashing lights and bleeps didn't alarm me and I could often distract myself from my various discomforts by taking an academic interest in what was happening to me and others.

In the high dependency ward and in the Liver Unit ward to which I next moved I had complete confidence in all the caring staff. For them I was a routine case. All the patients were being prepared for or recovering from similar surgery. The nurses detected the slightest wobble from the norm and treated us with sympathy and calm confidence. The medical team of consultants and junior doctors paid regular visits, as did the pain control team.

After four days I was moved to the comfort of the private wing; a generous bonus for a medical colleague. The peace and privacy and – not least – my own bathroom were very welcome. The downside was that I no longer had (or needed) the same close supervision. I had to judge for myself when to call the staff. I found this difficult, never knowing whether I might be distracting them from a needier patient.

Despite the high standard of nursing, I realised that the staff could not possibly have the same intimate knowledge of my condition as those in the Liver Unit. Mine was just one of the many wide-ranging illnesses and operations, with their own complications, with which they had to deal.

Luckily I was making a straightforward recovery so I did not feel alarmed just, at times, discomforted. My only real trial was persistent vomiting; I have always had this problem after any anaesthetic. But my tender 10-inch scar with its 24 clips, as well as the pull of various tubes meant that it was particularly uncomfortable this time. The vomiting continued for seven days despite the concerned attention of doctors, nurses and the use of a wide range of anti-sickness drugs.

Because I was on a private ward, I was allowed to have my flowers with me, which was lovely. Hygiene demanded that no flowers were taken into a general ward. But while there, my ever-increasing number of bouquets filled the window sills along the corridor to the Liver Unit and provided a wonderful scent if also a distinct reminder of the line up at a crematorium.

Once I was clearly on the mend Ronald returned home to man the garden and the telephone, to ready the house for my return and to compose the email bulletins. I was happy to be peaceful, just thrilled to be alive and relatively free from pain. I wasn't yet able to concentrate on any serious reading, which was frustrating as the pile of tempting novels and biographies grew by the day. Most of the time I was happy to daydream – reflection would be too grand a word – and to listen to music.

I did enjoy visits from a few very close friends including my brother-in-law Rob and his new wife Helen, the McDowells, Patrick Pietroni and my sister Felicity. Faith Hallet, a close friend and erstwhile colleague from the Multiple Births Foundation, was perhaps the most welcome visitor of all as she gave me the best present – a massage accompanied by a fragrant cream. This should be part of everyone's post-operative treatment. Again John O'Donohue writes on the value of touch:

> Touch communicates belonging, tenderness and warmth. . .
> when you are lost in the black valley of pain, words grow frail and
> dumb. To be embraced and held warmly brings the only shelter
> and consolation.

When stiff and aching all over, nothing can feel more soothing or reassuring. What with tubes and stitches, most of me was either too tender or inaccessible for Faith's administrations. But my feet loved it.

Eight days after my operation, I stopped being sick and could finally manage without an intravenous drip. My wound had healed beautifully, fit for a bikini, had I been many years younger. And then, just as the dressings were due to come off, my tummy was suddenly covered in huge blisters. An alarming and unattractive sight to me but dismissed calmly as a mild allergic reaction to elastoplast by the medical team. Although I knew it was of no serious consequence I was disconcerted by the deformation of my otherwise beautifully healing abdomen. Surprisingly so considering the relative triviality of these blemishes compared to what had gone on inside me – and might still be.

The disproportionate effect of trivial experiences, both good and bad, was something that was to go on surprising me over the months to come. It was as if I couldn't make sense of the bigger picture and therefore needed to concentrate on little problems, minor discomforts, which in the grand scheme of things are nothing.

With blisters settling, and the first meal after my operation safely retained I was told I could go home. I felt cowardly declining the offer (and the nurse's expectation) of a car journey home. Sitting in a bump-free chair for more than 15 minutes or so was uncomfortable. I knew that sitting in a car for 75 miles would be excruciating. As it was, on day 12 I travelled on a stretcher and was extremely grateful for the excellent driving and distracting stories of the cheerful two-man ambulance team. My hospital stay was over. That was the straightforward part; I had no idea what lay ahead.

12

Convalescence and Friends

AS THE AMBULANCE deposited me home, it felt as if a new and strange life was beginning; I felt like a visitor in my own home. Ronald had beautifully prepared the house and my welcome – as if he were a host expecting a special guest. For weeks to come, I was to feel like a guest, the receiver, in charge of myself but nothing more.

Our house could have been designed for the convalescent. From my bed I had a clear panorama of the garden through windows extending the whole length of one wall. From here I could see the valley beyond framed by the distant Black Mountains ending in Hay Bluff. The view was interrupted only by an eccentric array of Ronald's rather grotty birdfeeders, which tits of various kinds, chaffinches, nut hatches, yellow hammers and the odd woodpecker, shared relatively harmoniously with an expanding family of agile grey squirrels.

The newly converted conservatory with my chaise longue was only a few wobbly steps away. A trolley could be pushed right through from the kitchen to the bedroom and then into the conservatory without a single spill. Ronald was on call in his study next to the bedroom. Visitors could reach me through the conservatory without interrupting him.

My first day home Ronald had to go to an important meeting so Julia, my Cévennes walking partner, drove over to spend the day with me. This was the first of many happy times she and I spent together over the next year. Apart from preparing dainty morsels, her other task was to help the three young daughters of my secretary Jane Gardiner. By now there were well over 100 cards to be displayed. I didn't want the house to look like a hospital ward so we agreed that all cards should go into the conservatory. A memory I shall treasure is that of the girls decorating the conservatory under Julia's guidance. Not that they needed it. I know no children who are more imaginatively creative. Blu-tack and string were all Jessica, Lucy and Bethany needed to produce a colourful if eccentric art gallery mixing reproductions of old masters with the touching paintings of young friends and neighbours.

Another visitor on this first day was the community nurse, part of the General Practice team who gave me such wonderful attention throughout my convalescence. She carefully checked that my wound and I were doing well and that I had a good supply of dressings and medication. She also took extensive details of all aspects of my life noting whatever equipment and facilities might be required to meet all my needs and those of my carer. Had he all the support he needed? I was even given details of allowances available for carers – I didn't tell him about these as I feared he might prolong my time in the cared-for role.

Although I was doing well and had little pain, I was surprised, and disconcerted, by how tired I felt and was just glad to be at home, where it was peaceful. I looked forward to friends visiting later but not yet.

An unexpected post-operative side effect, rather than a complication or problem, had now developed: my sleeping pattern had changed. I have never given much thought to sleep as it had always been predictably sound and pleasurable. The only problem was that I had never been able to read in bed, so quickly did I fall asleep. I would then sleep deeply until I woke spontaneously and refreshed, ready to get up anytime after 5am, rarely later than 6.30. This had been the pattern throughout my adult life.

Apart from occasional jet lag, I could count on one hand the number of involuntarily wakeful nights I had had, and I had hated them all. Of course as a junior doctor I was often woken several times during the night. At such times, however, when duty was done I would go straight back to sleep. Now I was awake most of the night. Sleeplessness, like childlessness, has a negative connotation so I prefer to say sleepfree. Just as some people, although not myself, are happy to be childfree, I was quite happy to be awake during these nights. I found it a very productive time.

I would often wake at about 1am and spend three or four hours by the Aga with mugs of hot chocolate, reading or making jelly and chutney from the abundance of soft fruits and vegetables being picked by Ronald and unwary visitors during the daytime.

To my surprise I had none of the morning hung-over feelings that I knew so well when deprived of sleep as a junior doctor. Nor did I suffer from the night-time gloom and anxiety that sleepless friends and patients have described to me. As I had no heavy duties during the day, I was happy just to accept this new sleep pattern. From the start I rejected any suggestions of sleeping pills and have continued to do so.

On the whole this erratic sleep pattern has continued. It is a nuisance if I am away from home and must lie in the dark by the side of a somnolent partner. Apart from that, it doesn't worry me. I am happy to use the half hour or three hours for writing, reading or cooking. I usually then return to bed for an hour or more's sleep. Overall I seem to need less sleep than before my operation. Perhaps I am just expending less energy than I used to.

My train journey to Birmingham two weeks after my discharge from hospital felt like a major expedition. This was for an outpatient appointment with Mr Mirza. I took some trouble to dress smartly for the occasion and he would have been surprised by the pleasure his letter to my GP gave me.

> This lady on whom I carried out a Whipple's just over three weeks ago visited clinic today looking fantastic. She has made an excellent recovery.
>
> . . . histology has unfortunately come back as showing an ampullary adenocarcinoma that is lymph node positive (3:21 positive).

But the second part showed of course that my appointment had not all been good news. Indeed it was a disappointment as I told friends in the next instalment of our newsletter.

Convalescence and Friends

Quercwm Hospital Bulletin 6 August 2005

Dear Friends

At last I can do a little emailing on my own.

The standards of care at Quercwm Hospital are still rising and it may soon be awarded its fifth star, thanks not least to the input of so many generous friends. The freezer is filling rapidly with wonderfully nutritious chicken broth, fish stew, lamb casserole and chocolate cake. Nor is the psyche neglected – healing candles, wise First Nation CDs and a pile of improving literature.

Yesterday was the follow-up visit to Birmingham – my first journey of over 50 yards. The surgeon said my rate of recovery from the operation had been remarkable and we all agreed that this was attributable to the quite exceptional home nursing care. A second consultant and medical student were actually summoned to admire such a picture of health!

The main message from the visit was, however, less good than I had been hoping (if better than Ronald had feared). Although the tumour seems to have been thoroughly removed, there has been some spread of the cancer to just two or three lymph nodes and they recommended that I should consider chemotherapy – which I had hoped to avoid. But there we are and I know that several of you have had this without flinching.

I don't expect it will be so bad. It is not of course brilliantly convenient as there will be lots of treks to Birmingham hospital not to mention postponement of our bolder international travel plans. But at least we have discovered an excellent direct train from Hereford (which is only 12 miles from home by car) to Birmingham University with only a 500-yard walk to the cancer

clinic at the other end. I shall know more after seeing the
oncologist next Friday 12th.

Meanwhile we both send lots of love

Libby with Ronald

My second outing was pure pleasure. On a glorious clear August
morning Frances drove me up into the gorse-covered Radnor
hills of Wales. There Charles and Jane Williams greeted us with
carefully selected ice cream and other comforts as we looked
west, across a breathtaking vista of valleys and hills stretching
towards the Atlantic coast beyond. A timeless view and a
timeless drive. The intensity of the experience was the first of
several over the next year when I felt overwhelmed by the
beauty of the natural world, of my friends and the dread of
losing it all.

During these first weeks I was deeply touched by the care
and generosity of so many friends. Generosity not only in their
gifts but also in their time and thought. Each gave their own
special support, be it laughter, tears, chicken broth, smoked
salmon, chocolate, candles, massage, drives in the car, flowers,
smells, books, music, cards, letters or emails. Nor was the carer
forgotten, and our wine cellar benefitted.

I had many peaceful hours to myself. A golden opportunity
to read and no shortage of books, but I was disappointed how
poor my concentration was and it was all I could do to read
more than a chapter at a time of light novels such as Alexander
McCall Smith's *The No. 1 Ladies' Detective Agency*.

However I spent happy hours reading and rereading all the
messages in my cards, letters and emails. Many were moving,
others funny, a few tactless but all generous and loving.

Convalescence and Friends

For some, writing to me seemed to bring back long distant and sometimes deeply felt memories. I was particularly moved by the reflections in a letter from a friend of Bunny's who used to stay with us in York and later became a nun. I hadn't seen her for many years but she had heard of my illness through mutual friends.

The train stopped in York and memories flowed happily in of staying with you and spending time with Gran! As it pulled away north I glanced back and the Minster seemed to be riding slowly on the flat landscape like a stately ship. It seemed slightly unreal, yet in some other way more 'real' than anything else, like this train speeding by – so solid it stands. I've only come north about once a year recently; it's always a journey I feel engaged in very fully – a massive trek through memories and associations and stages of my life/journey.

Your journey too has had deep involvement with places – among them York and Yorkshire. And many joys and wonderful people. . . Dear Libby. . . Durham Cathedral has just sailed smoothly by with the same question – is it unreal or this train more so?

By now it must be clear to you, I don't know what to say, but simply want to write and post. Now we are gliding through Northumberland, and the landmarks of where I lived. . . I remember how strange it felt to leave, and how I questioned my perception/discernment/decision! I look over there now and ask what difference it would have made if I *hadn't* left.

Now the North Sea/Amble/Alnmouth flow by. My response surprises me [to the question] and I just think everything matters, with a quiet gentle intensity, in the present moment, wherever we are and whatever we do – and every moment and experience shapes who we are and are becoming.

Life is entirely gift, and also mystery, however much is revealed. But certainly whatever troubles and mystifies us there is a huge core of the acquired sense that 'all shall be well' and love is of the essence and does triumph over *everything*.

I was amazed, not only by the number of people from whom I heard, but also by the variety. Some I hardly knew, or had had no contact with for many years. I was particularly touched by the consistent thoughtfulness of Roy Strong. Although a close friend and neighbour he could have been more than forgiven for keeping his distance. Not only was he extremely busy, but it was only two years since his wife, Julia Trevelyan Oman, had died of pancreatic cancer. We had been privileged to be with them both during her final weeks and had admired the way they had coped so realistically and lovingly with their tragedy. For many months I received a weekly postcard – even two – from Roy. Each was carefully chosen with its own message and relevance. By the end I had a veritable art gallery of beautiful reproductions.

Inevitably some friends were more attentive than others. On the whole this was not related to the closeness of our friendship but to geography or to their own circumstances at the time. I know I give much better support myself if I have been in on a friend's crisis from the beginning than if I arrive back from my travels to find they are well into their journey of illness, bereavement or whatever and have already gathered a cohesive support group.

I also know so well how difficult it is to help friends when one is preoccupied with one's own worries or troubles. I felt sad that I was not able to give more support to our neighbours during the terminal illness of their lovely talented 13-year-old son. They were surrounded by supportive friends and the loss was more mine than theirs.

Compassion fatigue must inevitably be a problem for some. I would have more than understood if my own family had left others to look after me. They were all drained by the prolonged illness and death of my father and shattered by the death of Alice. Yet every single one rallied round once again.

I was particularly concerned for Sue Ramsbotham on whom I had leaned so heavily through our previous personal crises and illnesses. She had just given enormous emotional and practical support to a close childhood friend throughout an unduly prolonged terminal illness, culminating in giving the tribute at her funeral. Sue deserved a rest from her support role. I hesitated to even tell her of the new development in my life. In the end I wrote a brief note and said that I would more than understand if she would prefer to be spared the day-to-day involvement which she had always so generously given in the past. We could reconvene, I suggested, when I was recovered.

Needless to say she would have none of that and her messages kept me cheered up for many months. Her witty, forthright style is made for emails. She can say more in 10 words than most of us can in 50. I was actually glad we were 150 miles apart so that email remained our main form of communication.

By mid-August I began to enormously enjoy visitors. I could often receive them on the terrace or, if very hot, on the lawn in the shade of the catalpa tree. On wet days the bedecked conservatory served well. However, I was surprised by my poor stamina for even the closest friend. Within the hour, Ronald would rather firmly offer a tour of the garden, even to the least horticulturally inclined. I was embarrassed that many people would come long distances, some over 100 miles, for such a short time and receive only a cup of coffee or iced elderflower cordial as a reward. We soon restricted visiting to between 10.30 and 12.30 and from 3.30 to 6pm and a bossy answerphone message warned that even telephone calls were not welcome after 7.30 at night or between 1 and 3.30 in the afternoon.

I sometimes wonder how we would have coped in a pre-email era. It was our godsend. Ronald has never been keen on the telephone. Indeed, some of my colleagues were greatly relieved when I acquired my own telephone line so that they no longer risked the brusque, alarming to many, voice of my spouse. I was used to being the person who answered the phone in our home but now Ronald nobly, if unenthusiastically, took over this task.

But he was much happier, indeed very happy, responding to emails on his laptop. Each instalment of the Quercwm Bulletin generated a large 'postbag', which gave him encouragement and amusement. He spent many hours composing these news-letters, which in turn inevitably caused some MTs. We tended to disagree on the amount of artist's allowance permissible as well as how much personal detail should be exposed. I also worried more about imposing on busy friends who had more interesting and pressing matters to attend to than our domestic life.

However, judging by the insistent demands for more, there was no doubt that many friends enjoyed these missives. Others probably only read the first reassuring paragraph or skimmed through but seemed to like being kept in touch. Some, no doubt, were mystified by some of the humour, especially those less knowledgeable about the virtues of a wormery in gardening. (The welfare of the worms was often described in considerably greater detail than that of the patient.) Perhaps others were bored by them.

But we were sad that one close friend actually found the humour inappropriate and was concerned that Ronald may not be appreciating the seriousness of my condition. Nothing could have been less true. But for us humour is our lifeline. I can't remember us having an argument that has not been resolved in the end with laughter. I hope that, like my father, I can still be making and enjoying jokes on the day I die. As Ulla-Britt Linquist, the young Swedish TV reporter and mother wrote in *Rowing without Oars* just a few months before she died: 'Laughter is a deliverance. Disarming. It keeps danger at bay. Both aspects of a theatre mask: one happy, one sad. A fragile thread between tragedy and comedy[7].'

Ronald, naturally, did not want his valiant caring activities to go unnoticed. The emailed newsletter gave him chance to report on these and the temporary relief in store.

Many of you will be anxious about threatened 'burn out' in the carer. So you will be relieved to hear that that R & R for the carer is coming by convoy from York on Monday. Lucy and Lenore have had professional lifetimes in nursing. . . The task would of course be too great for one conventionally trained nurse alone.

Lucy Staples and Lenore Hill had been my colleagues during my

[7] Linquist, Ulla-Britt, *Running Without Oars*, John Murray, London, 2006

first paediatric job in York in 1968. Lucy was the ward sister and taught me more about looking after children than anyone. Both Lenore and I were new to the ward and equally nervous. Lenore was the junior staff nurse who later went on to great things, becoming the first director of St Martin's Hospice for children near York and the much-loved friend and support to many suffering families.

To their lasting credit, they managed to take over the kitchen and cooking with such tact that Ronald was not even tempted to advise, let alone criticise. They extended their duties well beyond the call of the patient – chutney making with surplus runner beans (of which there were many) and stocking the freezer with soft fruit.

During these early weeks some friends gave me Brownie points for courage. This gave me pause for thought. What they really meant was that I seemed quite cheerful, didn't grumble much (except to my poor carer) and had no difficulty talking about myself. Actually these are just the ways I found it easiest to handle my situation. I needed to talk, friends responded positively to my cheerfulness and this boosted my morale. My emotional well-being is enormously dependent on other people. My inner resources would, I fear, be very limited had I not the reassurance of knowing friends were always there when needed.

As they were for John Diamond, who so honestly wrote about this in his book *C – Because Cowards Get Cancer Too*. Like him, I could hardly feel sorry for myself after spending time in a cancer unit with people whose physical, mental and financial suffering was so infinitely greater than my own. And who may well not have the degree of support from family and friends that I have had.

Convalescence and Friends

I have always, even before I was afflicted myself, rejected bellicose words such as 'fight', 'battle' and 'defeat' in relation to cancer. They imply there is something to be conquered. Although I am sure attention to lifestyle and spirit may help, no amount of courage or bravery can necessarily bring about a cure. I prefer words such as 'coping', 'living' or even 'journeying' with cancer (although I have never come round to the 'befriending' favoured by some people).

Nevertheless I do think there may be useful parallels between cancer sufferers and soldiers on the frontline. Both find themselves in situations that are unexpected, uninvited and unwanted. My father, who was something of a Second World War hero, was interested in what constitutes courage and reflects on this in his wartime memoirs *Wool, War and Westminster*:

> I became interested in the subject of courage. . . I believe in the theory propounded by Lord Moran, Churchill's doctor, that each of us has a capital of courage upon which we draw and therefore expend. It is never easy to be brave but it is easier your first time into action and gets harder and harder as the campaign goes on. . . An individual's courage can vary in varying circumstances. When well led, among old friends, pride and self-confidence can make him brave. Thrown into battle after being newly posted to a poorly led unit in which he knows no one, he could emerge a less robust character.

There are times in my life when I have required courage. As a child it often took enormous courage to get back on my pony after a fall. It took courage to give the tribute at my father's thanksgiving service. He was a good public speaker and had been munificent in his (constructive) criticisms of my own performances in the past. And in both examples I had a choice to opt out.

With my cancer I have been given no choice. And my courage has not yet been tested. I have not had to repeatedly face the same ordeal. There has been a novelty about each stage. I have been well led by my medical team and have certainly been among old friends. Any suggestion that courage is needed to talk or write openly about what I was going through is far from the truth. I should have found it much harder *not* to talk or write about myself. An accusation of self-indulgence would be much nearer the mark. Actually the greatest test came when facing, and trying to keep cheerful through, the repeated blood tests and intravenous transfusions during the months to come. But for that ordeal, endurance would be a more appropriate word.

There are a few things I have done in my life of which I am proud. The handling of my cancer is not one of them. I am proud of being responsible for the first Parents of Twins Club in York, of establishing and directing the Multiple Births Foundation and perhaps most of all enabling some individuals to discover their potential and achieve more than they had dreamt possible. None of these actions were ones I needed to do or was called on to do. I did them of my own initiative, volition and with some determination. With my cancer, I have had few options and no great initiatives to take. I suppose writing this book may be the first.

Moreover I have felt unusually at peace with myself. As my father said:

In the war many people. . . felt more at peace with themselves than in times of peace. In war your conscience is clear. You know you are doing the right thing. . . . In peace you are lucky if you are confident that you are living to the best of your ability. In war your pride is at rest. You never chose to be a soldier. If you happen to be a good one, *tant mieux*. If you aren't, well you never chose to do this anyway.

With my new phase in life I knew I was doing the right thing. My overriding priority was putting what limited energy I had into following the doctor's instructions and doing all I could to facilitate my recovery. I was told clearly how to do it. No one asked me to make any difficult decisions. I was shielded from domestic or wider family worries. Any anxiety-provoking work such as writing, lecturing or symposium organising was on hold. I had time to concentrate on overcoming my cancer.

13

Six Months of Chemotheraphy

JUST OVER FOUR weeks after my operation Ronald and I went to meet the oncologist to discuss the question of chemotherapy and whether or not I should enter a trial currently being conducted in a number of cancer centres in the UK.

Until recently surgery was the only treatment offered for patients with cancer of the pancreas. Now if the primary tumour can be removed, there is hope that some kinds of chemotherapy may prevent or at least slow the spread of the cancer. This has yet to be proven, however. All types of chemotherapy have side effects, some of them nasty, some occasionally life-threatening. Before chemotherapy becomes a routine treatment for pancreatic cancer, it must therefore be shown that it is likely to do good, and more good than harm.

As there are so many other factors that can influence the progress of the disease in any given individual, a treatment can only be proved to be effective if it is tested by a randomised trial – one in which a patient is randomly allocated to one of two or more regimes. One of these may be a 'no treatment' regime. In the case of pancreatic cancer the trial is known as ESPAC – 3 (European Study for Pancreatic Cancer Trial 3. Adjuvant

Chemotherapies in Resectable Cancer). Its aim is to find whether extra treatment is better than surgery alone, and if there is any difference in effect between the two types of chemotherapy.

The oncologist carefully explained the trial and said that if I chose to take part I would be allocated randomly to one of three groups. The decision as to which of these three would be made by chance. The options were: being put on Gemcitabine; being put on 5-Fluorouracil (5FU) and folinic acid; or no chemotherapy at all.

Both the chemotherapy regimes involved drugs being infused through a vein. In the case of Gemcitabine the drug would be given once a week for three weeks out of four for a period of six months. With 5FU this would be given daily for five days, every fourth week, also over six months. Thus for both drug regimes there would be six courses.

The details of the trial were clearly set out on sheets for patients and ended with a list of the side effects: nausea, vomiting and flu-like symptoms were the most common. Mouth ulcers, diarrhoea, low blood counts and vulnerability to infection followed. I was relieved, and rather surprised, that hair loss was not on the list. But neither was tiredness, which turned out to be much my most debilitating side effect.

A central aspect of the study involved assessing how the disease or treatment was affecting one's quality of life. I would therefore be required to complete a questionnaire every three months during the study and at increasing intervals over the next two years.

If I elected not to enter the trial, I would be left with the choice of my care continuing in Birmingham but with no further active treatment. In the likely event of my cancer recurring then I would just be treated 'symptomatically', to reduce unwelcome symptoms as much as possible. Alternatively I could seek a specific form of chemotherapy elsewhere. I would be unlikely to find this on the NHS, and might well therefore have to pay for private treatment or to go abroad.

If I decided against all types of chemotherapy, I feared that I would be inundated with well-meant but stress-inducing suggestions as to how I could 'fight' my cancer myself. As it was, kind friends were already sending me books, newspaper cuttings and references to a huge range of cancer 'cures'. Some involved new drugs or extreme diet restrictions and supplementations or exercises, enemas and, of course, often international travel and huge expense.

I was in no mood for exploration and decision, to struggle to work out the possible value or otherwise of this huge range of treatments, diets or activities that might perhaps do some harm. I much preferred to be told what to do by a reputable oncologist who was working within strict guidelines.

We were given a week to decide which route we wanted to take. Before the end of the train journey home, I knew that I must enter the trial. Not to do so would have gone against my instinct as a doctor. I knew the long-term value of randomised trials to others, if not this time to myself. Perhaps an equally important and less altruistic factor was that by entering the trial almost all responsibility would be removed from me. I wouldn't have to think about choices or to seek out my own treatment and worry that, due to inadequate research, I had failed to find the best.

Within the trial I could see advantages in both the

chemotherapy regimes. The intensive single-week regime would mean that I would have a rest for three weeks. Life would be less disturbed by being out of action for a week each month than a day every week. However a 150-mile round trip to Birmingham on five consecutive days would be hard going but I didn't like the idea of spending the nights away. I would have shied away from spending evenings with even the most understanding friends and the thought of a B & B on my own was depressing. One visit a week would be less wearing but it would mean a greater interruption to life.

Just as I was getting back to near normal activities after my operation, the thought of going backwards was disheartening. So I had brief moments of hoping that I might draw the third option – that of no treatment. But realistically I knew this would be a blow. To do nothing goes against my nature. If I had no treatment and the cancer recurred I would find it hard not to say 'if only'. I might also feel that I had to take more note of all the suggestions of alternative therapy that had been showered upon me.

As I waited, the suspense mounted as to which regime would be my allocation. And I found myself, typically and pointlessly, planning the next six months around each in turn.

At this point I was introduced to Donna Smith, who was described as the 'research nurse'. She was much more than that. She was an information provider, morale booster and friend. If in doubt it was to her that I turned for the answer to every question, big or small. Not that she always knew the answer, but she would always know who would, and usually ask them herself.

I would have hesitated to disturb Donna with telephone calls even though we were all given her numbers, including one for her mobile. So I was relieved to find that she was a happy emailer. These messages were always warm and to the point.

I thought of Donna as my key worker. I had always believed strongly in the importance of families having key workers and deeply regret the decline of health visitors in that role. In my early days of paediatrics all families with young children expected to be in regular touch with their health visitor. She would know all members of the family and their home circumstances. They could turn to her for the smallest and largest concern. In my later years the pressures on health visitors had become so great that sadly they were often only able to respond to crises rather than nip in the bud some small problem that could otherwise have escalated.

Donna was like an old-fashioned health visitor. No question was too trivial for her. She checked whether I could drive myself the 12 miles from the station after my chemotherapy; when I could expect to be ready to set off for Australia after my chemotherapy was finished; when and what vaccinations were safe for me to have. She told me how to contact the dietician and whether the rules of the trial could be stretched to allow me to delay my treatment so that I could go to a friend's funeral in Yorkshire on a Friday.

When I saw Donna at the clinic she would always greet me, as she did others, and usually give me more time than I deserved. When she was under pressure she would say so and apologise for not being able to stay and chat. But she never ignored me. I was very struck by this feature in most of the staff, particularly the nurses. I never saw one try to avoid the eye of a patient as they walked through the crowded waiting area. I wish

I could say the same for myself. When you are running late and have much on your mind, it is so easy just to look the other way. The nurses would always greet patients they knew with at least a smile however busy they were.

Right at the beginning they asked me what I wanted to be called – by my first name, or as 'Mrs' or 'Dr'. I had no hesitation in answering 'Elizabeth' but I was glad to have been asked. I have seen elderly patients, unused to being called by their first names, feeling disconcerted by such familiarity from someone less than half their age.

My lot turned out to be the Gemcitabine regime, once a week for three weeks in each of six months. I was pleased. By now I realised that the practicalities of this would be the easiest to manage. The information was sent to my family doctor in a concise letter, ending 'All patients will be followed up in clinic every three months until death.' It was encouraging to think that I would be so well supervised. But there was a discouraging undertone. The clinic would get very crowded if many survived for more than a year or two. Little may the writer of the information have realised the impact it might have. There is a tightrope to be walked between clarity and unnecessary gloom. In contrast I remember one friend describing the relief when told that her mother would be followed regularly 'for the first two years', the first signal of hope that she might still be alive in two years' time.

My chemotherapy sessions started two weeks later and always took place on Fridays. The pattern was the same throughout with only minor variations. I would leave home just before 7am to drive to Hereford station. There was no question of Ronald driving me to Birmingham because of his leg.

Anyway, there was no point in him wasting a day as well as me. Many kind friends offered to be chauffeurs. But I preferred to go by train. I could read or sleep without worrying about anyone else. It gave my lowering morale some satisfaction that I was still in charge of myself. And with a Senior Railcard it was amazingly cheap!

I would catch the 7.42 train direct to University Station in Birmingham. Then there was only the short walk through the university and hospital gardens to the main Queen Elizabeth Hospital. The cancer clinic was on the ground floor just near the main entrance.

By 9.15 I had clocked in, put my blood-test forms on the pile and settled down with a good book in a comfortable chair in the still relatively empty reception area. After some minutes a firm call of 'Elizabeth' would ring out and Ann, the phlebotomist or blood taker, would usher me into the blood-taking room. The blood tests are vital. The results decide whether the body has the resilience to accept another dose of chemotherapy.

I dreaded the first time they were to take blood as my veins are notoriously difficult to enter. But I had never met a defter blood taker than Ann. For the first few sessions she was in and out in a jiff and with no more than the 'little prick' described so euphemistically, but inaccurately, by my previous blood takers.

Even in the later more difficult times the discomfort was compensated for by the lively stories from Ann. Whatever the ups and downs of her own life, she told her stories with such humour, which was bound to distract the most anxious patient. Indeed two of my accompanying friends asked to come in for the next instalment.

However, over the months these sessions became an

increasing challenge for Ann and the chemotherapy nurses. Towards the end of my chemotherapy it could take over half an hour and many jabs and bruises, to get the small amount of blood necessary for the test and the cannula inserted for the transfusion. This was no reflection on the skills of the operators, only on the well-recognised paucity of my veins. When I was going through infertility treatment involving daily blood tests it was finally agreed that it would be better if I took my own blood – from the back of my foot. As a junior doctor on the neonatal ward my Group O Negative blood could sometimes have been very useful to my little patients – if only my colleagues could have got it out of me.

After my blood test I was given the result straight away. Over the months the suspense increased. If the haemoglobin level was too low I might need a blood transfusion. It did fall low enough to make me feel more tired and sometimes breathless, but never low enough to need a transfusion. The platelet counts were also of importance. If they got too low there could be serious risk of bleeding in or from any part of the body. Although I had an impressive array of bruises from the blood-taking attempts, I was spared the bruising all over the body that some people suffer.

More concern was focused on the white cell count. The normal range for a white cell count is $4.0 - 11.0 \times 10^9$/L. Chemotherapy drugs suppress the activity of the marrow including the production of the white cells. If the white cell count gets low there is a risk of serious, even life-threatening, infection.

The trial had rigid criteria. If the total white cell count was below 2.5 the dose of Gemcitabine was reduced to 75 per cent and if the count was below 2.0, the chemotherapy was cancelled altogether for that week and then resumed at 75 per cent of the previous dose. As I waited for the result I often felt ambivalent. The thought of not having to go through the uncomfortable transfusion followed by the days of exhaustion was very attractive. However, I argued to myself, to miss one of my treatments might just be the crucial difference between killing off the last cancer cell in my body and allowing one to remain hidden only to multiply later. And anyway to turn round and go home felt an awful waste of a journey. In fact, only once in the six months was my treatment actually cancelled. After that visit my dose of Gemcitabine was reduced.

Once I knew my blood-test result I would take the report through to the chemotherapy department for a cheering welcome from the receptionist and a place in the queue for treatment later in the day. The pattern was different on the first Friday of each month's course. On that day I would first be weighed and then have an appointment with the consultant oncologist or one of her registrars. They examined my tummy, admired my now inconspicuous scar, shared my regret over the (luckily, now fading) scars from the elastoplast allergy blisters and never failed to say they were pleased with my progress. As my weight was holding near the eight and a half stone mark, they were less concerned about my erratic bowel habits than I was.

These clinic appointments gave me the chance to discuss some of the questions on my mind. I was still intrigued to know whether my BRCA1 cancer gene was the cause of the cancer in my pancreas. This they could not answer. Pancreatic cancer is much less common than cancer of the breast or ovaries so it is unlikely that enough cases could be gathered at the moment to find out. Not least because most BRCA1 candidates in the past would have died from cancer of the breast or ovary before any cancer in the pancreas had had time to show itself. Perhaps by having my own ovaries and breasts removed, I had in fact allowed the gene to be active in producing an even more life-threatening type of cancer.

No one could tell me, nor can they now. And I don't dwell on this thought. Nor should I. I tell myself that I may well have had many years of good health that I would not otherwise have had. Bunny was only 43 when she developed cancer. I was 63.

Although the five-year survival rate for pancreatic cancer sufferers as a whole is very poor – only about 2–3 per cent – I was told that my own odds were considerably better. Because my tumour had been fully removed and there was no sign of the cancer having spread beyond the local lymph nodes, my chances of survival had now improved to between 30 and 35 per cent. Not marvellous but a great deal better. However, it still made sense to be prepared. I therefore asked what signs or symptoms I could expect should my cancer recur. The doctor was reluctant to answer this, encouraging me not to think about it. This was advice I would be unable to follow.

At my Liver Unit follow-up appointment later in the day I had a helpful talk with Mr Mirza. He said that I was most unlikely to have a recurrence during the six months of chemotherapy nor within six months of its completion. The highest-risk period was in the 12 months following that. Usually the symptoms are fairly non-specific, such as weight loss and general tiredness. He said, thanks to the operation, I was unlikely to develop either an obstruction of the bowel or jaundice. I was greatly reassured to hear this. I had hated the malaise associated with my jaundice and had watched the agony of a bowel obstruction for Bunny.

Most of the doctors were sensitive but, perhaps inevitably, they occasionally hit the wrong note. 'Goodness doesn't time fly' was not the right response to the news that I had now had three months of chemotherapy. 'Well it may for you' was my chilly retort.

After my clinic appointment I would wait until my Gemcitabine had come up from the pharmacy. Even when I had no clinic appointment this rarely arrived before lunch. I was unperturbed. I had no other plans for the day and was never bored in the clinic. I was fascinated just to see the clinic in action. Cancer is not limited to any age, social or ethnic group. We were an odd mix. A few looked tragically ill. Most of us looked pretty good, and it was often difficult to tell who was the patient within the – sometimes large – family groups. Short hair or no hair at all was often the telltale feature. Unlike most hospital clinics most patients felt at home here. If you regularly spend many hours idling away the time in one place, you get to know it and the various people who help you there quite well, from those who gave us drinks from the volunteers' coffee shop, to the receptionist, and the counsellor in the Cancerbackup room. One was free to browse through all the Cancerbackup booklets and other literature without disturb-ance but the counsellor was always discreetly in the background if wanted.

Whether my chemotherapy arrived from the pharmacy before lunch or after, I was usually able to keep 1 to 2pm free for a picnic lunch with friends. This was the highlight of my day and sometimes allowed me to positively look forward to a day at the clinic. The nurses were wonderfully accommodating, sometimes hurrying my treatment through but, more often, just postponing it until my guests had left. Once it was as late as four o'clock to allow me to go with my friends to the under advertised but delightful Barber Institute Art Gallery, less than half a mile from the hospital.

Apart from my book, the only luggage for the day was a bright yellow cold bag, chosen so that it could be easily identified by my friends. Should I be tied up in a treatment room it would mark my camping spot for the day. In this bag was lunch for anyone who might be joining me. I tried to have a treat menu. The standard one included quails' eggs (a useful size), goats' cheese with lettuce and smoked roast salmon sandwiches, grapes and chocolate. Some enterprising friends brought welcome additions such as soup, cake and flapjacks.

It was a wonderful chance for reunions with friends from the past. But the greatest bonus of all was that it allowed me continuing contact with my 18-year-old niece, Catherine, who was at school only 10 minutes' brisk walk from the clinic. I was touched by the regularity with which she came when her life was so full with A levels and other school activities.

Two people, Julia Gregson and Frances Hancock, actually came over by train with me and joined me for the full works, including the session with the doctor. Julia, herself a novelist, had been encouraging me to write a book about my experiences. I welcomed her suggestion that she should come and see this new and strange part of my life about which I would be trying to write. We talked non-stop throughout our train journeys and most of the day!

After lunch, with coffee in hand, I set off for my chemo-therapy session. This took place in a large open-plan room just off the main reception area. In it were 10 or so treatment bays each with two chairs, a chest of equipment and space for the stand to hold the various bags of fluid that were to enter our veins. Nearly all of the candidates had a relative or friend with them. Some were there for several hours. Others, like me, were luckier and got it over within an hour.

Of all places within the Cancer Unit, the chemotherapy room might be expected to be the least cheerful. Many of us would not be alive next year and the staff must have been constantly saddened by the death of people whose journey they had shared and cheered on over many months, sometimes years. Despite this the atmosphere was one of calm bustle and cheerfulness.

The chemotherapy room was manned by a team of very experienced sisters and staff nurses. As treatments were confined to the administration of highly toxic drugs, the responsibility could not be given to junior nurses or medical students. Quiet confidence exuded from our carers and suffused us, the patients. I am sure they must have had their worrying moments, even scares, but these were always well concealed. Instead there was always a good balance of concern and laughter. I trusted them all and never minded which of the team was to care for me that week. They clearly all respected each other too and there seemed little competition. There was a rule that after three failed attempts at inserting a cannula they should hand over to a colleague. This was always done without resentment – a much healthier approach than that of some persistent junior doctors I have known who wouldn't give up!

In addition to the Gemcitabine, which would be left to drip into me slowly over half an hour, the nurses would give me two other injections to reduce the side effects such as nausea. These had to be given quite slowly. (One of them could cause a weird pin prick sensation in one's bottom if given too quickly – I gather for men it can have a more exciting effect!) So there was always a time for chat with the nurses as they sat with syringe poised. Over 18 sessions there was a chance to get to know several of them quite well. They each had their own interesting lives that I enjoyed hearing about. We all looked forward to the arrival of a first baby and the weekly reports of its progress. I was very interested in the dissertation of another on different types of palliative care and the plans for an exotic holiday of a third.

Several of them asked about my own paediatric work. They managed to respect my professional life while treating me as a patient. I was grateful for that.

When my Gemcitabine infusion had finished, I was free to go, and often did so at some speed to catch the next, only hourly, train to Hereford. Unfortunately, by now, the train was either full of school children, or an hour later, with Birmingham commuters. Either way the rail company had not catered adequately for the numbers and the train was already tightly packed by the time it reached the University station from Birmingham. It remained full for the next half hour, until Worcester. This was my least favourite part of the day but luckily the after-effects of my chemotherapy didn't strike for at least 24 hours so it wasn't too bad.

I usually arrived home in good spirits, being one lap nearer the end of the marathon. For the first months the pattern was predictable. I would feel fine on the Saturday, but knackered on the Sunday – an extraordinary exhaustion I had never experienced before. Usually when tired in the past, even after the most gruelling days and nights on duty, I could struggle on as long as necessary. Now I couldn't summon the will power or strength to do more than shuffle from my bed to the chaise longue in the conservatory. It was as if my reserve tank of energy had emptied. Often I would just retreat to bed and curl up like a fetus, sometimes for hours.

On these days I was neither depressed nor particularly unhappy, just utterly drained. Ronald accepted this extraordinary change in me with equanimity. He left me in peace, manned the telephone, and offered drinks and nourishment with no fuss. He would sometimes lie beside me. Never had his presence felt more reassuring. I could have felt very lonely. I often thought of the many who did not have such support and wondered how I would have coped without him.

Looking at us as a couple many people would assume that of the two of us, I would be the more natural carer. I belong to a 'caring profession' and I perhaps appear more patient than Ronald, who tends to get going a bit in an argument. They would be wrong. Had I been a natural carer I would have trained to become a nurse rather than a doctor. And I never took readily to my caring role towards him.

I am probably more patient than many as a listener, always being interested in other people and their problems. But when it comes to practical caring my boredom threshold is very low and I am bad at hiding it. That combined with impetuosity and clumsiness makes me about the last person anyone would choose as their carer. Even as a server of breakfast in bed, Ronald is more careful and thorough.

Six Months of Chemotherapy

After his major surgery for cancer and consequent leg problem, I had taken on the role of carer to varying degrees over the following eight years. Not always graciously. This last year has caused an upheaval in our caring roles.

We both have a tendency to be 'over helpful'. We frequently try to improve each other's ideas and plans. This has been an accepted, if sometimes maddening, part of our relationship. On the whole we are each strong enough to resist the alterations with which we don't agree and to accept, if grudgingly, the improvements. However Ronald seemed to realise that this old pattern wouldn't work when the balance of strength became unequal.

From the moment I became ill, I cannot remember Ronald ever trying to impose his own views or to alter my plans. He also turned out to be extraordinarily good at detecting and responding to my fluctuating moods. He knew instinctively that I was vulnerable, that I could easily be undermined. Even if he thought my poor stamina meant a day trip to London or giving another lunch party was unwise, he never even intimated this. When I then collapsed in a heap at the end he never said 'I told you so' nor worse still the dreaded patronising question of the past 'And what lesson have we learned?' Sometimes, perhaps I might have liked a cautionary word or hand, if only to be able to blame someone else for a plan's failure.

During my chemotherapy, I know that some people thought I was trying to do too much. Some even said or implied that Ronald should stop me. But managing to live a life with some semblance of normality was what kept me going – and gave me hope that I might return to it when all the treatment and disturbance was over.

At times Ronald must have been irritated and frustrated. He would watch me entertaining my guests animatedly, knowing that he would have to cope with the wet rag afterwards, a drab and often tetchy companion.

Ronald has many good qualities but patience is not one of them. His threshold for mental boredom is considerably lower than mine. And he is sometimes not good at concealing it. He can be confrontational and daunting in discussions to those who don't know him. But while I was so evidently unwell, he remained amazingly tolerant. So much so that the occasional return to his usual irritable self was a relief – if only because I knew then that he thought I was getting better.

By the Monday after my chemotherapy I was feeling better and by Tuesday I was almost back to normal and would be happy to resume many ordinary activities, even go to London for a night or two. During the two weeks between courses of treatment we would take advantage of the predictable good times and invite friends for the weekend, or go off for a night or two in Wales. Twice we did a two-day Eurostar trip, first to Bruges, then Lille.

Planning treats was one of the best therapies during these low periods. Many of the plans have still only been undertaken in our dreams. My plan for a Carers Lunch Party took effect just after the New Year. I wanted to say thank you to six people who had played very special parts in my recent journey. I felt enormously reassured that this team now knew each other and would be there to support Ronald and me through whatever might lie ahead.

For the first few months of chemotherapy there was a regular pattern. As time went on life became less and less predictable. I never knew how long the tiredness would last, sometimes right until the next treatment. My bowels, which had been troublesome since my operation, became even more erratic and I had quite a lot of abdominal pain. I sometimes had symptoms that scared me. Perhaps the more so because my medical knowledge fuelled my imagination.

Although I had been told that a recurrence of the cancer was very unlikely during chemotherapy, the slightest deviation from the norm made me fear the worst. One morning I woke up to find the whole room swirling round me – an attack of vertigo that ended five minutes later in vomiting. Disturbing as the experience was, it was nothing compared to the fear of the cancer that must have spread to my brain. It never happened again. It was probably nothing to do with my cancer. Another worrying symptom that would appear several times a week in the early months was an acute breath-stopping pain under the right side of my rib cage. I imagined cancer invading my liver.

After various consultations the combined opinion about this, with which I was happy to concur, was that the pain was probably caused by some damage done during my operation. This was reassuring. It was not life-threatening and was likely to gradually disappear. It did.

These occasional symptoms were scary but nothing compared to the many side effects I could have had and didn't. I was lucky. Very. I have known friends on chemotherapy who have had horrid mouth ulcers, skin rashes, difficulty in swallowing, loss or distorted taste and, of course, loss of hair. I was ashamed at the intensity of my dread of hair loss. It should surely be of small note in this life-threatening journey. Initially there was more hair on my hairbrush and in the shower plug than usual and I feared worse would follow. But I never lost any serious amount and I was hugely grateful. The only significant loss of hair was under my arms. My armpits were denuded for many months and only needed shaving again after a year. A small but definite bonus.

I have had a number of friends who have carried their temporary baldness with aplomb, either using it as an excuse for exotic headgear, a wig, or just apparently comfortable in their new Yul Brynner image. I would have hated that and could never have remained as cheerful and elegant as my sister Felicity with her array of fine silk turbans.

Apart from being embarrassed had I lost my hair, I didn't want to be labelled as someone with cancer. As it turned out mine was probably the easiest outcome. In a gathering I did not stand out as having anything physically wrong with me. But anyone who knew me well could hardly fail to notice that my shape had changed, so that served as a reminder to treat me gently.

For the first time in my life, I had difficulty in maintaining my weight. In the past I have often tried to lose it. Now I had to take in calories whenever I could. As often happens after major bowel surgery, despite feeling hungry, I could not manage a large meal. I would quickly feel bloated and uncomfortable. But then I would soon become hungry again. I took to 'grazing' small amounts throughout the day and much of the night. I often had hot chocolate and porridge in the early hours of the morning. Always on hand was a tin of finger shortbread and bars of dark chocolate together with a jar of nuts. All three came in a plastic box in my handbag whenever I left the house, together with an elegant Regency-style pill box containing my pancreatic enzymes. Without them, much of the nourishment would be wasted. For someone who has always loved their food but tried to resist eating it, it was exciting to be able to eat chocolates whenever I felt like it. But it was also frustrating, or more accurately, boring to have to keep thinking about what would cause indigestion. I had always had an iron constitution; I now longed and needed to eat but found it hard to eat enough without discomfort.

I have always had a voracious and somewhat indiscriminating appetite. I could enjoy almost anything, marmalade and honey being the eccentric exceptions. Now things changed. I had strong internal messages as to what would be good for me and the messages varied from day to day. It was as if my disturbed digestion had knocked me off my metabolic balance and specific replenishments were sometimes needed urgently. One day I would only feel like carbohydrate and would consume large amounts of porridge and rice. On another I craved fats as in cream, yoghurt, butter and cheese.

Throughout the six months my fellow traveller Sue Norrington and I kept in close touch, by telephone, email and, when possible, by meeting face to face. We explored our pains and experiences together. My training probably gave me more insights into the physical side, hers certainly to the psychological. I found her thoughts on how her body and soul were adjusting to the new situation very helpful. This is part of an email she sent to me:

About the pains – I have them too from time to time.

Those who have also had big abdominal ops tell me that they've had them too – often continuing for quite a long time.

What makes sense to me is that the whole of that area has been severely traumatised and bashed about quite a lot while the op is being done, though I find it difficult to distinguish the muscle pain from the post-op internal pain – and then the chemo. I think I'd feel much happier if someone could sort that out for me.

I've been thinking today how much the whole of me has been in shock. I've kind of allowed for the mind and emotions to feel like that, but now I think the poor old body has had the same sort of response, and from time to time it's just very painful for it. I think it must be such a huge shock for the whole person, body and soul, and I feel as if I am gradually allowing myself to feel that now, rather than having the reflex healthy instinct to get on with it, survive it and get better. I do find myself, especially yesterday and a bit today, kind of dreaming around the place, as if something is quietly going on in my unconscious, doing the work of readjusting to the post-op situation, where an awful lot has happened and changed. Perhaps it is a coming together of the whole person again after a bit of it has been stuck in a horrific limelight. It's so difficult to feel whole when one bit is the focus of everyone's attention!

I so agree with her. And I particularly resent the part of the body that it has to be. Any other bit of my anatomy would have been preferable to the bowel. I hate to have to think about it, let alone talk about it. I seriously considered not writing about it. But not to do so would be to omit the most time-consuming and all absorbing preoccupation of the last 12 months. It is however the hardest section of the whole book to write and I only do so with great reluctance.

I find the whole vocabulary of ingestion, digestion and excretion difficult. To stick to medical terminology – faeces, evacuation – removes all emotions, and there was a lot involved. To use the doctor-to-patient terms of stools and bowel movements seems euphemistically inappropriate and hardly portrays what I really felt. As it is a long time since I had to care for patients with bowel problems, I don't normally have to talk about the subject at all so have had little cause to explore current vocabulary: shit, crap, poo. . .

My bowels have caused me pain, discomfort, anxiety and much embarrassment but worst of all they have often stopped me thinking of anything else. Whenever I was alone, my thoughts would come back to my bowels, however hard I tried to concentrate on more attractive and interesting subjects. By day I was constantly aware of their presence and they were often responsible for my wakeful nights. It was only when I decided to write this book and started composing in my head that I finally managed to divert my thoughts from my innards. Had this book never got further than a failed attempt it would still have played a major therapeutic role in my recovery.

The first problem was the discomfort and, sometimes, pain. I was constantly aware of the activities within my abdomen. It was as if I could track the journey of each bolus of food or air (of which there was a great deal) on its journey along the 22 feet or so of bowel coiled within my abdomen. Sometimes it would get stuck and I could feel the bowel contractions straining to move it on. The colic could take my breath away.

My evacuations, as my doctor called them, were frequent, often six or more in the day. They were often explosive, always offensive. I dreaded this when in other people's houses and had a small air-freshener aerosol in my handbag. The problem was increased because often it was difficult to flush the faeces away in one go. When the bowel is not absorbing normally, the residual fat in the faeces makes them float and it can take three flushes to clear the loo. Difficult when at the theatre with the interval bell ringing and an impatient queue outside. How long can one monopolise the only loo in a café? And I could really only stay overnight with friends who could provide the luxury of a loo to myself.

In fairness, most of these problems were in the morning, so I tried to avoid early-morning appointments. If I couldn't, then I would often take a precautionary anti-diarrhoea pill and wear a pad. I never had a major accident. I would have been mortified. But it made me realise how agonisingly difficult it must be for those who are more infirm or who do not have the facilities or choices that I did.

I shudder too to think how insensitive I may have been to some families in my clinic. I had failed to appreciate the extent of the practical and social problems faced by the whole family when there is a young child with coeliac disease or cystic fibrosis, both are diseases that stop a child from absorbing food properly. Many of these families lived in small houses and would have had only one toilet, often within the bathroom. No young child would have taken the precautions I could to avoid accidents, or to prevent the smell pervading the house.

As a result of my weight loss and lack of exercise over many months, my muscles had seriously wasted. My skin was hanging loose and I was pathetically weak. The 200-yard walk from our house up a cart track to the road felt like a mountain climb. The table tennis that had been very much part of our life was too demanding. When I tried to play I resented being so badly beaten by Ronald when I was used to nail-bitingly close matches. I hated the look and feel of my body. I knew I should do something about it but was finding it difficult to summon the energy to do so. Somebody then suggested yoga.

I clearly wouldn't have the stamina for a group class but someone was recommended who specialised in teaching yoga to people who are incapacitated in one way or another.

I had known Jenny Bullough for many years but we had never known each other well. I never expected that we would. She is 10 years younger than me, dark haired, petite and warmly demonstrative. And she moves with a delightful combination of poise and agility. She wears clothes from the parts of the world, such as India, that most inspire her. Jenny had many qualities that I admired but also found daunting. I assumed we were unlikely to have a lot in common. I was quite wrong. She has been a huge strength and help to me but we have also developed a close friendship that culminated in a happy week together at a course on psychotherapy and the arts.

I knew nothing of yoga but I soon learnt that, in addition to the focus on breathing, the two main ingredients were physical exercise and meditation and that it was up to me to decide what balance of these two I wanted. Apparently younger yoga practitioners usually concentrate on the physical aspects and then over the years, meditation tends to take up an increasing role. I had come for the physical aspect. We worked on that basis.

However, as time went on, I have been amazed by how much I came to value the peace and focusing of my mind induced by the exercises and the very specific breathing that accompanies them.

Over the months I have worked through various exercises which have increased in complexity and the strength required. But always I was told not to push myself. During my chemotherapy, when my energy levels were so variable, I had exercise options for good and bad days. I aimed to do my 20-minute regime each morning in our visitors' room which, like our own bedroom, looks out at the Black Mountains but has fewer distractions in it.

In the early days I often failed to summon up the necessary energy and several days might be missed. Now I rarely miss a day, except when I travel, and look forward to the monthly session with Jenny when I am given a new and slightly more demanding programme. By most standards I am still on the nursery slopes. But there is no doubt that I am more sprightly and my muscles are much less flabby – and I really enjoy it.

I also enjoy the single sheet personalised programme that Jenny produces for me, illustrated with evocative matchstick figures that inspire me to greater activity and agility.

Regular walking is the other obvious way for me to exercise. But I have never been a keen walker, and no dog or other reason has forced me to be so. Indeed circumstances have been against it. Ronald always thought walking a pointless pursuit unless we could return with a sack of leaf mould or armfuls of logs. For me this detracted from the walk. So we rarely set forth together, even before his leg problem and certainly not after. But now I am welcoming the chance to walk, partly as it is one of the few exercises, other than yoga, that I can manage, partly for the chance to explore our beautiful neighbourhood but mainly because it allows me to continue a new friendship.

Frances Hancock had supported me through all the worst periods. Our friendship had blossomed into what was inevitably an unequal relationship. We both realised that our relationship would be different once I had recovered. But whatever happened we both wanted it to continue. As our patterns of life and circle of friends overlapped relatively little, this would need organisation – it wouldn't happen automatically. A regular walk was the answer.

Despite the discomforts and unpredictability of my bowels and the frustrations of my poor stamina, I was surprised how good my spirits remained. Although my sisters and I have been spared the severe form of manic depression experienced by my mother and Alice, I have always tended to have mood swings. There are times when my highs provide the energy and early rising which give me a reputation for enthusiasm, hard work and productivity. Less attractively, certainly to Ronald, are my impetuosities and over-talkativeness that tend to go with this phase. We have a code for when I am getting high at dinner parties.

During the lows I have much less energy, become more anxious and am less early to rise. I of course dislike these low times but always know they will pass and have learned to wait relatively patiently for them to do so. Although I am never aware of the low times being triggered by outside events, I naturally find them harder to cope with when other things in life are going less well.

I was therefore enormously grateful to be spared a low throughout this last year. I have been constantly surprised by my continuing good spirits, which are nothing to do with stoicism or courage, only with how I happen to feel. That is not to say that I have not at times become weary and disheartened by my bowel eccentricities – 'bowel growel' as one fellow sufferer called it – or sometimes fearful of what may lie ahead, but I have never had that deep down, inexplicable low that I have known in the past.

I have no idea why I have felt so cheerful. Whether it is physical factors such as a change in my hormones that are responsible, or the reduction in external stresses combined with the constant morale boosting of friends, I don't know. There was no doubt too that I was being held in the hearts and prayers of so many dear friends and neighbours, not least by those in my own village of Vowchurch. The objective effect of such a safety net of prayer is not one I can ever know or even guess. I can only be deeply grateful to those who created it.

Whatever the reason for my resilient spirits, it is a most welcome side effect of the otherwise horribly unwelcome happenings of the last year.

Even when we are in calm waters Ronald too can have low spells. Yet through this year he, like me, rarely seems to have had these mood swings – or perhaps he has hidden them from me. Although he has always been as ready to cry as to laugh with me, he has tended to let me be emotional when I needed to be and has rarely showed his own anxieties and depressions.

I was so self-absorbed during the early months of my cancer that I am sure I often failed to respond to Ronald's feelings, or was probably not even aware of them. He is blessed with many friends as well as a loving sister and brother to whom he could have talked. I don't know how much he did. I suspect not a lot. I couldn't help feeling that this was a time when he especially missed having no children. I am sure it would have helped to have a son or daughter to share the emotional load.

My last chemotherapy was on 10 February 2006. I had of course been looking forward to this moment for six months. But the relief was inevitably tinged with a feeling of loss. I was no longer going to be the focus of such attention, no longer would I have the security of seeing people with whom I could share the smallest worry. I knew the telephone line was open 24 hours a day and that I could return to the clinic whenever I wanted. That was not the same as the reassuring thought that I would have weekly contact with people who cared and understood my illness so much better than anyone else could.

Having had my hand held for the last eight months, I was now setting off on a journey on my own. A journey that may end in a few months or continue for 20, even 30 years.

But of course I was not on my own and few people could have had more people to travel with them.

For some time Frances had suggested that I might like to join her for a service. Now seemed the time. On 2 March 2006 we set off on a Pilgrimage of Hope and Healing. The plan had been to go to the church of Evencoyd high in the Radnor Hills. As it turned out our plans were thwarted by an unseasonably snowy spell. We chose instead the nearby church of Gladestry, which had the advantage of not only being more accessible but warmer.

As we set off the threatening clouds parted to reveal a bright blue sky and the snow-clad landscape glistened in the sun. At the church we began with a warm welcome from Marion, the priest. Frances and I were then left to share together a beautiful service starting with the Intention:

Death may live in the living and healing rise in the dying for whom the natural end is part of the gathering and of the harvest to be expected.

To know healing is to know that all life is one and there is no beginning and no end.

And the intention is loving.

Margaret Torrie

We reflected, prayed and anointed each other. The service ended with me reading Thomas Merton's prayer:

My Lord God, I have no idea where I am going. I do not see the road ahead of me. I cannot know for certain where it will end. Nor do I really know myself. . .

I will trust you always, though I may seem to be lost and in the shadow of death I will not fear, for you are ever with me, and you will never leave me to face my perils alone.

We then knelt quietly listening to the slow movement of Beethoven's Piano Concerto No. 5, Op. 73 'The Emperor' played by Alfred Brendel.

14

Moving On: A New Project

Dear Friends and Colleagues

I write to tell you of a change in my life. It means that with many of you I will no longer have the active working relationship that I have enjoyed for so many years in collaborative studies, on committees, advisory and editorial boards and symposia platforms. I plan to take no further active part in the world of multiple births once my present commitments are fulfilled.

I went on to explain why and my plans for writing this book and ended:

My work with colleagues, parents and twins themselves has been endlessly stimulating and I shall miss it very much. What I have learnt over these rewarding years will greatly help me in this new project and of course my interest in twins will always remain. Needless to say, I hope to stay in touch with all my many friends in the world of twins. In particular I shall remain in close touch with Jane Denton, the current director of the Multiple Births Foundation.

I sent this letter on 11 February 2006, the day after I finished my chemotherapy. On the train returning from Birmingham, I had made the sudden, perhaps impetuous, decision to change the direction of my life. And I knew it was right. For 32 years multiple births had been my overriding and passionate concern. The time had come to move on.

And no better, if uninvited, opportunity could have presented itself.

The timing too was right. My interest in twins had started five years before the first IVF baby was born in 1978 and from then on there had been a steady increase in the number of twins in the UK and in all developed countries, due to the common practice of transferring two or three embryos at a time in an IVF cycle. Finally in 2006 the Human Fertilisation and Embryology Authority recommended that the best way to give IVF was by transferring only one embryo to the womb at a time, thereby almost eliminating the risk of twins. I no longer had the role of trying to convince infertility specialists that twins should be avoided, whenever possible. The great majority now agreed and for those who didn't, government regulations would dictate their practice. My work in this area was over. In the areas of paediatrics, counselling and bereavement there was still work to be done but there were many others to carry on the work.

Thus the letter was sent to colleagues with whom I had worked in the field of twins and triplets over the past 30 years. These particularly included members of the Multiple Births Foundation, the Twins and Multiple Births Association and the International Society for Twins Studies as well as many individuals who in one way or another had helped me in my work over the years.

I expected one or two to respond warmly. I was overwhelmed by the numbers, many from overseas. And also their generosity amazed me.

The director of a multiple births organisation in the US wrote:

> You need not worry about abandoning the twin world. Your twin work is not over, not by a long shot. . . not even if you never write another twin-related article or give another talk. Your indefatigable efforts on behalf of multiples continue to have positive ripple effects all over the world.

From a child psychiatrist in London:

> It has been an enormous privilege and pleasure interacting with you over the years and I know that I have learned a lot from you. For that, very many thanks. You have been a real towering pioneer in the world of multiple births and it has been extremely important to have them put on the map in the way that you have achieved.

A paediatrician in London:

> I have learnt much from reading your writings and listening to your lectures over the years. . . You have made a fantastic and matchless contribution to the subject, and always without pretension or pomposity.

A professor of nursing in Canada:

> I am pleased for you that you can pass the torch of multiple births on to others. You have given so much, inspired so many, and lead the way for so long. It has been a tremendous commitment and you have excelled. How wonderful that you can soon begin your reflections in Bali with sand between your toes, the fragrance of jasmine, and conversations with gracious people. . . I know that whatever direction you choose to take, the journey will be right.

Here was a response from a mother and doctor in America:

> You have been a warm, encouraging, helpful presence to many parents, and to me in particular as I sought to cope with my twin son's stillbirth and to educate others with my own work. Thank you for all you have done in a remarkable career to date, for so many parents of multiples internationally.

And from a friend and fellow traveller, an infertility specialist:

> I do not believe in going into elaborate philosophical considerations about it, but as somebody who has undergone a similar experience I nevertheless feel entitled to wish you all the physical and moral courage that I know in my bones to be needed in such a situation. Knowing you, I am certain that you will once more prove to be the bravest of fighters that you are. Unfortunately, I cannot do better than to wish all the best to you and also to Ronald.

Moving On: A New Project

What I hadn't expected were suggestions that our previous collaboration could be continued but in a different way:

> It is wonderful that you are going to put your personal and professional experience to good effect by writing about BRCA1 and the choices presented to individuals and families. We would be very keen to be supportive. Just tell us how we can help. We could do some polling or have an event to bring people together in a seminar around your project. We often have people contacting us about whether they should have breasts removed – just in case.

> If you need assistance or other people's experiences in some way for this new project, let me know. I come from a family where everyone three generations back has had cancer, but it hasn't been possible to identify a mutation for anything. That is also a problem because it leaves us in a kind of limbo.

> I have been struggling – in the past, but especially recently – with (serious) genetic problems in the family and I'd be only too glad to share my thoughts and experience with you. . . we might become colleagues again, albeit in a different branch of medicine.

Others telephoned me and had further suggestions of how I might collaborate in research projects, particularly to do with the counselling issues surrounding genetic testing and Pre-implantation Genetic Diagnosis.

I felt some of the old excitement for fresh projects. But I cautioned myself. Life was different now. My energy was limited. And so may be my time. The essential must come first. And that was to get down on paper the story I wanted to tell. I knew I had been blessed with all the requisites for a story that could be helpful to others. I should be deeply disappointed if I didn't have the time to tell it.

However tempting the other projects, I couldn't be diverted. Once the book was finished, then I could spend the rest of my life, short or long, pursuing the increasing number of fascinating trails that were being offered. Just now I must get on with the story. Especially as I wasn't sure how easy I would find the writing. For the first time I should be writing very personally, and I am not a professional writer. I am all the more conscious of that as I am surrounded by writers in my family. My sister Felicity was a journalist before she became a literary agent and both she and my husband are authors of several books.

Ronald has always been invaluable in his editing of my scientific papers, chapters and textbooks but he doesn't usually boost my confidence while he does it. 'How can you make something that is so interesting seem so dull?' was his response when faced with the draft of one of my early papers. At least the story this time has the potential to be a bit less dull than the transfer of proteins across the placenta.

It also had, I knew, the potential to help me through a difficult time. I have often suggested to bereaved parents that they should write not only about their baby or child who had died but also about their own feelings. I had seen how therapeutic this can be. I knew it could be to me too. Just the thought of the book helped even before I had written a word. As John Diamond said a few months before he died of throat cancer:

> There is no doubt that knowing that one day (provided there is a one day) you may write about what is happening to you is a solace not on offer to patients unblessed by a similar instinct. For a writer, nothing is ever quite as bad as it is for other people because, however dreadful, it may be of *use*.[8]

There were some other small ways in which I felt I could use my experience. As a medical student I had received excellent teaching on the diagnosis and treatment of diseases. Little, however, had been taught about the emotions and feelings of the sufferers. Over the years I have gradually learned about these aspects from my patients, far more than from any lecture or textbook.

Yet, as I approached retirement, there were still huge gaps in my understanding and knowledge of psychological medicine, not least in the field of cancer. Had there not been, my own responses to my illness might not have been such a surprise to me. Not that I expected there to be any single pattern of reaction to cancer any more than there is for bereavement. But at least I could have known more about the possibilities.

I was therefore eager to share my new-found wisdom with any student doctors, nurses or social workers prepared to listen and was disappointed that there were none available. Especially as I and my many fellow sufferers and their families had more than enough time to give our carers tutorials while waiting for or having our chemotherapy sessions.

Meanwhile I had some things to tidy off in my twins work. I offered most of my books to the Multiple Births Foundation,

[8] Diamond, John, *C: Because Cowards Get Cancer Too*, Vermilion, London, 1999

my many reprints to various colleagues writing at the moment. The paper shredder burned out and had to be replaced. Fortunately the best of my 6,000 photographs and slide collections had already been transferred via a scanner to CDs.

There were a few remaining commitments that I had agreed to before the onset of my illness. I gave my last lecture in Melbourne and completed my task as guest editor of a special edition on Multiple Pregnancy for the journal *Early Human Development*. I had been involved with this journal for many years first as assistant editor and then as a board member. It was a fitting finale to my writing on twins and I was gratified by their generous editorial tribute, even if it did read like an obituary.

15

Bonuses

I have heard it said often on cancer wards that the best gift anyone can ever receive is to believe for a short time that you or your family is under sentence of death but then miraculously to be reprieved. Because the understanding and self-knowledge you acquire while peering into the abyss can form the basis of a life that is so much more meaningful and profound – if only you could get the chance to live it.

So wrote Lindsay Nicholson in the *Guardian* on 27 May 2006.

I agree with her. I have no doubt at all that if I survive I shall regard this last year much more as a gift than an ordeal. It has been an experience, however unpleasant at times, which I shall never regret. If I have only a short time to live, I am deeply grateful to have had this time.

Over the last year each day has been precious in a way that I have never before known. I wished that I had learned earlier the wisdom of this Ancient Sanskrit poem:

Look well to this day
for it is life
the very best of life.
In its brief course lie all
the realities and truth of existence.

For yesterday is but a memory
and tomorrow is only a vision
but today, if well lived, makes
every yesterday a memory of happiness
and every tomorrow a vision of hope.

Look well, therefore, to this day.

A death sentence from cancer for an adult is, I believe, far less dreadful than it would be from many other diseases. Death does not take us by surprise, nor does it surprise our friends and family. Given the choice, I would choose cancer over any sudden death. Preparations can be made. Sufferers are given time and hence so many gifts they might never otherwise receive.

Few people with cancer nowadays suffer severe pain, even if the numbers are still more than they need be. Pain can usually be controlled to allow the sufferer and his or her carers to treasure each day and to give each other comfort and pleasure, indeed for some, untold happiness. Certainly Bunny had this, and her dying wish 'that love should grow' was amply fulfilled.

Few cancer patients have frustrations with communication, so common in those who have had a stroke, for example. Nor the indignities of relying on others, sometimes for years, for feeding, washing and toileting as with motor neurone disease and other muscle wasting or neurological diseases.

I think it can often be easier too for those left behind. Fewer friends feel shocked or guilty. Fewer will have regrets of omission or negligence. They have had time to prepare, to complete unfinished business and to sort out any misunderstandings or grievances. They can say goodbye. My sister knew when the time had come for a final farewell to a close friend and she made it clear that that was it. She did not see them again.

I have lasting regrets over friends who died suddenly or where I had just procrastinated, failing to visit in time, or to say goodbye. My closest and lifelong friend died in her fifties. I still have to forgive myself for not talking as I and perhaps she would have liked during her final illness. I was under pressure from work and from our own family illnesses. But that is no excuse and the opportunity can never be recovered. The thoughtfulness and regular contact over the last year from her daughter, my god-daughter, is hugely appreciated but reminds me of my own neglect.

I cannot think of a single close friend of mine who would now carry such a burden. All can and should feel that they have given me more than I could possibly deserve or have expected.

Friendships, new, renewed or strengthened come high on my list of bonuses. The reviving and enhancement of so many friendships from the past has been a surprise and delight. These include friends from school, university and my years in Yorkshire, as well as from more recent decades. The only problem now is that I of course want them to continue. When I was convalescing, there was no problem as I had no other priorities. Now, if this book is to be completed, I must however reluctantly reduce the number of meetings for coffee, lunch or whatever.

In the last year of his life I remember my father saying to me that one of the great bonuses of getting old was one's increasing capacity to love. He was particularly moved by the depth of love he felt for his grandchildren. I don't now believe this was related to old age, but rather to the fact that he knew he did not have long to live. I have the same feeling now. Talking recently to a friend who knows she is dying of cancer we agreed that we felt 'an infinite capacity to love'. In the past, perhaps subconsciously, I had felt that 'loving' had to be reserved for partners and close relatives. That there was something shocking about loving too many people.

There have been some new friendships where there were small hurdles to overcome. True friendships need to be reciprocal but inevitably some relationships during this time were unbalanced. In the past, I suppose, I had more often given support than received it, particularly to anxious mothers or to those desperately trying to become mothers. My good fortune and particular professional background had tended to put me, if anything, in the role of care-giver. Now I was the receiver. I was not used to this and sometimes found it disconcerting.

Another bonus from cancer has been my reduced level of anxiety. When there is a possibility of death the problems of life, however great or trivial, loom less large. Now when things go well I feel as happy as I ever did. When they go badly, I definitely suffer less. I would love to be able to say that I have now relinquished useless anxiety but that would be an exaggeration. But I certainly don't waste nearly as much emotional energy on it as I used to. The most conspicuous example would be cooking. In the past giving a lecture to 500 people would give me much less anxiety than preparing a supper party for eight.

I have never enjoyed cooking and my more honest friends would probably say that they haven't particularly enjoyed my efforts. The only way to survive at all was to keep repeating the same dish from my limited repertoire until it was at least safe, even if it wasn't a culinary triumph. Once conquered the same dish would be produced with regular monotony. One loyal friend still teases me about my hare pâté phase, which appeared at every meal I produced when we both lived in York.

As we have always enjoyed seeing our friends and having them to stay, this ongoing anxiety over cooking has been a major handicap and a cause of great irritation to Ronald. More than once he has suggested we stopped entertaining altogether if the alternative was living with such an agitated partner.

Suddenly and inexplicably I am enjoying cooking. Particularly surprising as I can't myself eat much of what I cook. Or perhaps that's the explanation. I am even enjoying experimenting and am no longer so disconcerted by failures.

On a lighter note, there have been other bonuses. In similar circumstances each of us would find our own. Mine might seem odd considering the wide spectrum of opportunities that I could have grasped but didn't.

I have always been clumsy; kinder friends call it impetuosity or even enthusiasm. Our china breakage rate is probably higher than that of many families with young children. It was therefore always clear that I should never be a ballet dancer or a mistress of petit point. As a physical coward, high diving boards, mountain climbing and skiing, other than on the nursery slopes, were never on my wish list. I would have liked to paint and to be more artistic; I regret my poor memory and inability to recite a single poem. However I had gradually come to accept that all these challenges were beyond my reach and, by my seventh decade, had more or less come to terms with most of my deficiencies.

Acceptance did take longer in some areas than others. I found particular difficulty with those in which one or both sisters excelled. Memory was one of these. A lasting wound was inflicted when I was six.

My mother, an enthusiastic and persistent encourager, had taken weeks teaching me 'I Have a Little Shadow' for me to present as my Christmas piece to the family. With great apprehension I stood behind the curtain on the window-seat 'stage'. When revealed to the gathered audience I managed to stumble through the poem. The applause was more for effort than achievement. From the back of the room my tiny sister Felicity – and she was very tiny even then – piped up, 'Now I'll say it.' Lifted on to the window seat, she confidently performed the whole poem, word perfect.

There were two failings, however, with which I still had not come to terms. The first was my figure. All my life from a chubby babyhood I have been larger than I would have wished. I have never been seriously fat although I do look a very odd shape in some photographs aged 16 when billowing organza and hooped petticoats were briefly in fashion – at least in some parts of Yorkshire. During my adult life I would always have been happier to be a stone lighter. Never, despite repeated struggles and a range of absurd diets, did I manage to lose an ounce more than seven pounds.

A loss of two and a half stone has given me enormous

satisfaction and a figure whose elegance is way beyond my wildest dreams. I have always had a roundish face so the loss does not make me look gaunt, I am told, just very well, and improved by the loss of the double chin. I am astonished, indeed rather ashamed, by my current vanity. I rejoice in the words used by friends that have never previously been applied to me except in irony. 'Slender', 'slim', 'slight' are manna to my ears.

But recently 'skinny' brought me up short and for the first time made me realise that any further weight loss would no longer be a bonus. I now try hard to add a few pounds. But old habits die hard and each time I go on the scales I have to remind myself that to have lost another pound is *not* a good thing.

Even my mastectomies and subsequent implants have at last come into their own. Until now I had been able to find little compensation for so much pain and disfigurement. I have now found it. Whereas sudden weight loss in most women in their sixties would result in unattractively drooping breasts and a near flat chest, my implants mean that I remain surprisingly well endowed with no danger of the slightest droop.

The second failing was my singing, if it could be called that. This was acknowledged as a handicap to me and even more to others very early in my life. As long as I can remember I was told that I had inherited my mother's and grandmother's (non) singing voice, whereas Felicity and Bunny had our father's singing genes.

Although not an every-Sunday-church-going family, hymn singing was a major ingredient of our childhood. We regularly made long car journeys. Every Friday evening, we would have a two- to three-hour drive from Halifax in the West Riding to our farm near the east coast and back again on Sunday. Copies of the English hymnal were kept in the car pockets and my father, Felicity and Bunny would vigorously sing hymns for much of the way. My mother remained silent and I was only allowed to sing the 'Amen'.

When I went to secondary school all hopes for my singing career were abandoned and I was told that I need no longer attend the singing class, to the relief no doubt of classmates.

Despite all this discouragement I have always loved singing hymns and often do so when driving on my own. However in church, unless surrounded by very loud singers, I would mouth all but the lowest pitched hymns. I looked forward to the rare occasions when we had 'Eternal Father strong to save. . .' Over the years I have shared my sadness with my musical neighbour, Sue. She has always claimed that with the right guidance and encouragement (almost) anyone can sing. There was no reason why I shouldn't. I never believed her.

However, early this year, I suddenly decided to give it a try. I asked Sue to find me an especially gentle teacher. She found the perfect person. Joyce is a retired school teacher, the organist in a nearby parish, still a teacher of piano to some of the village primary school children and leader of the adult singing group. Joyce and I agreed from the start that she would treat me as she did her six-year-old pupils. She gave me daily exercises but told me on no account to let my husband hear me sing for at least three months. Wise advice. Ronald is by nature an encourager but has always been the opposite over my singing – self-preservation being a stronger instinct even than compassion.

Joyce is an unqualified encourager. Never before had I been told that I was 'absolutely on the note', and when a whole line of the hymn was said to be so, my joy was unbounded. Any wavering was attributed to unnecessary anxiety, never inability.

As I write this I am on the Welsh border at the Champernowne Trust week on psychotherapy and the arts. Each morning there is a half-hour singing session for the 60 participants with vigorous rounds on many of the regular favourites.

In the evening a smaller group, the 'Six O'clock Singers', gather for more sophisticated singing in preparation for a performance on the final night. I would never have believed I could have had the courage to join this group. . . but I have and I am loving it. My fellow singers are much too kind to tell me if they are enjoying it less.

One poignant favourite, written and composed by Jane Mayers, a former director of the course, inspired the title of this book. It is 'I Sing the Life':

I sing the life that is born in all of us,
Ours to use the best way we can.
I sing the death that is yet in store for us
Linking back to the place we began.

The paths we travel are often in shadow
But words are lanterns to guide our feet
And the joy of friendship and peace of solitude
Help the myth and the meaning to meet.

We tread the labyrinth of our being
To reach the shore on the other side
We feel the wear and the grime of our journeying
Each alone, with the thread for our guide.

16

Relinquishing the Invalid Role

MY CHEMOTHERAPY FINISHED on 10 February 2006. On 6 March we set off for a month in Australia via a few days in Bali. I was leaving as a battered convalescent. I intended to return with full vigour, eager to start a new phase in my life.

Australia was the natural destination: a country we both love, in which we have many friends and one where the chance of gastrointestinal upsets is fewer than in more exotic rivals. I had spent a year in Australia as a newly qualified doctor 35 years before, having come out as a cargo ship's surgeon, fortunately untested. Since then I had often returned for conferences and lecture tours, always extending the trips to see friends and explore new parts of the continent from Darwin to Tasmania, Perth to Cairns and, in New Zealand, from Auckland to Milford Sound.

Perhaps over-complacently, neither of us was anxious about the journey. We were used to taking risks. Ronald's bad leg had toughened us and he had survived septicaemia in northern Brazil. I have an eccentric love of flying. Perhaps it's the pleasure of being looked after and knowing that I am safe from any outside contact. I had often felt sad when even the longest and most uncomfortable economy-class flight finally landed.

This time we took the journey more comfortably and gently than usual, with a first break in Bali where we were enchanted by the people and their art and strengthened by five days of sun, swimming and massage. In Australia we were welcomed by medical friends in Darwin, and gradually recovered from their generous entertainment on the new North–South 'Ghan' train (named after the 19th-century Afghan 'cameleers') which took us the 2,000 miles to Adelaide in 48 hours.

From there we went on to Melbourne and Sydney, catching up with friends from all periods of my life: recent ones from the International Society of Twin Studies, then those from when I worked in South Korea in a mission hospital, and then from my original year as a paediatric resident in Sydney, and even with a fellow St Thomas's medical student, now a senior consultant psychiatrist in Sydney.

The highlight of the trip was an evening in my aunt Helen's flat that overlooks Sydney Harbour and its opera house. Helen, now in her nineties, had three younger generations at her flat, including her great-grandchildren, five- and three-year-old Lilly and Felix. Thanks to Helen having been tested and found to be free of the cancer gene, their parents know that these children will never need to worry about BRCA1.

True to my planning nature, I had decided I would arrive home from Australia fully recovered. I did not want to go back to the stressful life of the past but to a life of my choosing, to be able to do what I wanted. It was not as simple as that. On my return to England, although my spirits and most of my body did feel restored and indeed in good form, my stamina was not as good as it used to be and my unpredictable bowels remained a serious handicap.

I was still too frightened of being caught short to risk any meeting or serious activity before 11am or so. If I had to travel early, I would wear a pad for safety. Even later in the day, things could go wrong and Ronald got used to requesting a not especially needed coffee in the nearest café as I rushed in search of a loo, often thoughtlessly well hidden.

I resented this restriction to my life but more than that I was disappointed; I so wanted to get on with my new life. To all but my closest friends, I tried to appear fully recovered. Everyone told me how well I looked so they had no difficulty in believing it.

My emotions often got confused. One moment I was determined that everyone should think I was now well, in which case they could rightly think that I didn't want to be asked or reminded that I might not be. The next moment I was surprised, almost resentful, that so-and-so hadn't asked me how I *really* was. My friends and family just couldn't win.

Although Ronald was endlessly patient in listening to my muddled thoughts, I needed help that was less emotionally involved.

I am blessed in having a wonderful range of friends who are good listeners, many of them trained to be so. Many would have allowed me to talk for as long as I wanted. But the greatest help of all came from three with whom I had regular assignments: Patrick Pietroni, Frances Hancock and Jenny Bullough. I looked forward to these meetings; before each of them I could think about which particular muddled feelings most needed airing. I didn't have to pretend there was any other purpose to our meeting.

With these three I felt a safety described so aptly by Dinah Mulock Craik (although often ascribed to George Eliot):

> Oh, the comfort, the inexpressible comfort, of feeling safe with a person; having neither to weigh thoughts nor measure words, but to pour them all out just as they are, chaff and grain together, knowing that a faithful hand will take and sift them, keep what is worth keeping and then, with the breath of kindness, blow the rest away.

Before this current illness, I had been in buoyant health. I rarely saw a doctor, other than for the routine blood pressure check before my next HRT (hormone replacement therapy) prescription, which I had taken since my ovaries were removed 13 years before.

My only other medical encounter was with my plastic surgeon. Once the complications of my mastectomies had settled, it was agreed that I should be reviewed annually. As this appointment hardly felt a priority in my expanded scheme of hospital visits, I had postponed this year's visit for some months, until after my return from Australia.

When I finally went up to the Harley Street clinic one sunny spring afternoon, I did so with confidence, looking well and expecting a brief but encouraging visit. Not so. As an artist might look at a failed canvas, so did he look at my chest.

My breasts have never been appendages of which I was especially proud. I have not spent much time looking at their reflection in the mirror, certainly not since their experiences of three years ago. I was therefore taken aback by my doctor's expression and his comment about lopsidedness. He invited me to look in a large mirror. Now that he had pointed it out I could see that he was right. The left was much smaller than the right and also had a large bubble on its left flank. This, he said, was 'like a tuck'.

But he assured me that all was not lost. I had the convenient valve under my arm through which he could inject some more saline and blow the left one up a bit. He thought this might also remove the tuck. I agreed that this should be tried and I felt myself being gently blown up like a Michelin woman. I now eagerly awaited my next look into the mirror. The expression on my surgeon's face should have cautioned me.

My left breast had indeed blown up but only in one half. Apparently scar tissue had restricted the inflation of the other. Not only was the breast now an even odder shape but the two nipple tattoos were facing in different directions – like someone with a severe squint.

Far from improving matters, the process had clearly worsened them. Again the little valve came in handy and the saline was removed. I returned to my previous shape with nothing more to show for my visit than a plaster and a mutual agreement that I would only return if I had problems. New problems.

By June 2006, my energy was returning and I was of course grateful to be alive but I really wanted more comfortable and predictable insides. I therefore wrote to Mr Mirza:

Dear Mr Mirza

As I approach the anniversary of my surgery. . . I would welcome the chance to review my likely long-term health should

I be spared a recurrence of the cancer. Although everyone thinks I look wonderfully well (probably because of my new elegant figure) I still get quite a lot of discomfort, bowel unpredictability and I have difficulty in maintaining my weight, with consequent reduction of stamina, limited diet and some social inconvenience.

It may be that I must just accept all this and be grateful to be as well as I am but I would value your advice. . .

A friendly reply and an appointment followed. Mr Mirza was as helpful as before. His verdict was that I looked very well but I shouldn't have been having these bowel problems. He and the dietician both felt that there should be something I could do to improve matters. He thought that I wasn't absorbing food properly and that was why I wasn't gaining weight and why I often had such an unpredictable start to the day.

Mr Mirza recommended that I treat my pancreatic enzymes 'like salt' and not like a medicine and try taking a lot more. They also thought that by limiting my diet (i.e. avoiding fruit, salads and the like) I could well have altered the 'flora' and therefore the digestive environment in my gut. I should therefore try reintroducing them.

He ended by warmly telling me how well I had done this first year but that the second, the next 12 months, would be the real test. I'm not sure he need have been quite so candid. It's much easier to be honest to oneself (which I think I am) than have someone else state the facts so baldly.

But on the whole I really appreciated his candour if only to reinforce my resolve to make the most of every day. We had an interesting discussion on telling patients about their illness. He believes that all should be fully in the picture. Indeed he said that in his particular unit there is no option. With so many people sharing the care, including six consultants, several registrars and other junior doctors, it would be impossible to keep track of what a patient and their family had been told were it not the whole truth.

I am still unsure. Perhaps part of me still belongs to the 'paternalistic' group of doctors who tell the patients what they consider is best for them. I hope not. But I do sometimes think that I have told patients more than they wanted or needed to know. Of course any question should be answered truthfully, but I am still uncertain whether it is always right to offer patients bad news on which they can take no action and is of no benefit to them.

I remember as a more junior paediatrician I had a policy of always telling parents if I heard a 'murmur' in their baby's heart despite knowing that the majority of these 'murmurs' were innocent and would just disappear in a few weeks or months. I told them because I believed that I would tell them so sensitively that I would allay any possible alarm. I flattered myself. I soon learnt that however carefully and reassuringly I gave the news there would always be some parents who would be deeply upset. Through a mutual acquaintance I might hear that this same healthy baby had a life-threatening heart defect and that the whole family was distraught.

What I am quite sure about, however, is that there are very few times, if any, when a patient and their family, should not be told if they are dying and clearly entering the terminal phase of their illness. I shall never forget the beautiful 32-year-old sister of a close friend of mine who was dying of cancer and she didn't know it. Or at least it was assumed she didn't as she had never been told and she never spoke of it. How isolated she must have felt. What agony not to be able to discuss with her husband the future plans for her two young children. I hope this situation would never arise nowadays.

I followed Mr Mirza's advice on dietary and enzyme adjustments. A definite change followed. My bowels became much more predictable but with a price of feeling bloated and no doubt looking several months pregnant most of the time. I at least now had a choice of discomforts and hopefully, over time, might be able to work out an optimal balance.

Another big step on my road to recovery and normality was the annual week-long course on psychotherapy and the arts run by the Champernowne Trust. The summer course is now held at Buckland Hall, a retreat centre in the Brecon Beacons National Park in Wales.

As chairman of the trustees for over 30 years, the trust and the many friends within it had always been an important part of Ronald's life. For many years I felt sad that it was a part that I didn't share. It was a world in which I would love to have felt comfortable but feared I wouldn't. I thought I would find the public expression of feelings threatening. I was unfair to it; I never gave it a chance.

It was only when I was invited to be one of the annual course speakers that I risked the plunge. That was in 1995. Since then I have returned four times as a participant. I always enjoyed the courses and got a lot out of them but regretted that I couldn't completely relax and take the personal risks that others seemed to do with such ease. I perhaps compensated by never quite relinquishing the caring role. Never had I been confident enough to risk some of the activities that I knew I might be bad at, such as the singing or a solo performance at the do-it-yourself evening.

Ronald and I returned to the Champernowne Trust in July 2006. This time it was a quite different experience for me. There was no longer doubt where the balance of care lay. I was 100 per cent a receiver. As many of the old friends were here again, I had a wonderfully warm welcome and throughout the week was given a quite undeserved degree of thoughtfulness and care. I was deeply touched.

The summer course at Champernowne has a standard format which has evolved over the years. The options start from 7am when a party would set off for a swim in the River Usk. At 7.30 there are half-hour sessions of meditation inside the Hall or t'ai chi on the lawn, which is bathed in breathtaking early morning lights from over the Brecon Beacons. After breakfast we all meet for morning singing. Following this an invited speaker talks on some aspect of the week's theme. This year the theme was 'Body and Soul'; last year's had been 'Significant Transitions'.

Painting or clay modelling is available in studios that are open and welcoming day and night. I took advantage of the clay studio. Here you can choose a lump of clay and do whatever you like with it. Some use it as an opportunity for artistic creation, others as a chance to explore their feelings. For me it was the latter. I was determined to try and come to terms with my bowels in the hopes of relinquishing my current humiliating and boring preoccupation. After a gentle creation of long coils of clay as the smooth bowel of my past I then took a second lump of clay and had great satisfaction in kneading it fiercely into the coils with kinks, constrictions, dilations, knots and explosive expulsions that represented the present. The third lump turned into a pyramid of smooth coils almost in the form of an offering or sacred mound.

My second series focused on my cancer and the unknown. In the head of a large question mark was a spikey ball representing cancer that was blended with a heart. From it in one direction was a curved radiation of enlarging cancer 'balls' and in another a radiation of enlarging hearts until the two again met. Once I had taken a photograph of it I smashed it and scattered the fragments in the garden. It was no doubt simplistic and unprofound by Jungian standards, but it was for me a small step on the way to learning to live with my new insides.

Two-hour workshops are on offer during the afternoons. This year's choices were drama, music, writing or movement. I had always chosen the movement workshop under the inspiring leadership of Nina Papadopoulos, a dance therapist, and was set to do so again when the news was broken that she had bronchitis and her workshop was cancelled. A replacement voice workshop was offered as an opportunity for those who had always wanted to sing but thought they couldn't. It was clearly made for me. And, it seemed, for several others. However, it also turned out to be an opportunity for others to enjoy a favourite pastime. Our leader, Hilary Fisher, seemed undaunted by this incongruous mix.

Hilary is a warm vivacious redhead with a wonderfully expressive face. Now an inspiring performer and singer, she has had many struggles along the way which she shared with us. Such were the obstacles that she had overcome that, had I been

30 years younger, she could almost have convinced me that I too, with a little effort, could become an opera singer.

Hilary was not concerned with achieving a choral performance from us but rather that we each should find and use our voices to their very best potential. This involved all sorts of antics that did not come naturally to me. We were all challenged to improve the quality of sound produced by increasing the volume of our pharynx. Sticking out the tongue as far as it would go and then singing at full but controlled volume was apparently the way to keep the sound connected to the body. A fly on the wall would have got the giggles, as certainly did some of us, at the sight and sound of 'Amazing Grace'.

When it came to the obligatory solo performances, we all seemed as nervous as each other but were each enormously encouraged by the great improvement that Hilary convinced us she could detect, be it in the volume, pitch or quality of our voice, in our deportment (we were to imagine our sternum suspended from a helium balloon) or in our muscle control.

Entertainment after supper varied. On the penultimate night it was do-it-yourself. Singers sang, musicians played their instruments, mimicry, mime and dance followed. Ronald sang his perennial Cockney pickle song as well as reading some Dylan Thomas. In the past this was an evening in which I enjoyed being a member of the audience and would never have dreamt of performing.

This time I told a light-hearted anecdote about inappropriate counselling and read 'Look Well To This Day' (page 223). I was touched by the number of requests for a copy and to hear from two therapist friends that it was now pinned up on their office wall.

For me there were many moving and poignant experiences during the week but perhaps the most treasured was the early morning swim in the River Usk. Several friends had encouraged me to do this. Their enthusiasm combined with their concern for my safety meant that the descriptions of the route to this idyllic swimming pool varied from a three- to four-minute gentle walk along the river bank to a 20-minute hard climb over a hazardous path with potholes, stiles and many a root or rock to trip over. Fortunately one gallant friend promised to carry me if necessary. So I joined the four-car convoy at 7am.

Surrounded by mountains bathed in the morning light, the site was a treat whether for swimmer or riverbank dreamer. A pebble beach and huge rocks on the banks and in the river created places where one could recover from exertions or just watch the birdlife as well as the swimmers. The rocks also created waterfalls, and in one place there was a diving spot into a nine-foot pool. In parts the current was strong, providing a challenging exercise for the energetic and a wonderful free ride return for the less so.

I was carried away by the beauty and joy of this experience and probably used more energy than I had since before I was ill. As I reluctantly left the water, Jenny Bullough was there together with others to catch and cosset with towels and a hug. I felt so overwhelmed both physically and emotionally that it was all I could do to reach a rock without fainting. Tears welled up as I was overcome by the beauty of this life and my own frailty.

17

How Truthful Have I Been?

I RECEIVED THIS letter from Patrick Pietroni in October 2006:

Dear Libby

I've read the chapters about your illness and am replying to your request for 'comments'.

You have managed to capture the factual scenery of your family history as well as your own personal journey with immense skill. I could find no error of 'fact', which you asked me to look for. You have written your story in an exciting and 'what happened next' style which is easy to follow and enjoyable to read. You camouflage your medical expertise with aplomb and avoid patronising comments, which you do anyway. Your close friends will recognise honesty, reticence and dignity and be well aware that you tell it as it was and is.

However your undoubted positive approach to the challenges you have faced and are to face could be seen by a reader who does not know you as a bit too rosy a description of your experience as a patient. Were you never angry, depressed or frightened? Were the doctors, nurses, receptionists never abrupt, rude or uncaring? Were none of your friends tongue-tied, unsympathetic, unable to find the right words? We are not all as sensitive as you! I know as a GP of 40 years that many patients of mine facing the challenges you face, have not been able to respond in the way you have and they have often had a very uncomfortable, painful and miserable time.

This may be a little unkind to say but one of the more helpful responses (so the research suggests) to being given a diagnosis of cancer, especially one with a poor prognosis, is denial. If I didn't know you so well and read your book, I would wonder about your response, not to say that it was wrong, on the contrary. But if you are writing a book as a patient and as a doctor you owe it to your readers to at least debate and interrogate yourself as to the possibility that your positive responses may be a coping defence against less comfortable feelings. Again can I reiterate, even if this is the case, the research suggests that it is as good if not better, in terms of prognosis than the other responses such as depression, anger or acceptance.

Written with much appreciation and admiration for the joy you bring to all who are privileged to know you.

love Patrick

Patrick's letter was of course written as a friend as well as a medical colleague. My strengths were no doubt given greater prominence than they deserved and my weaknesses less. Nevertheless I think he is right, that up until now I have coped pretty well. Better than I would have expected. I have never felt out of control, desperate, paralysed by fear or anxiety. I swore no more than usual and never screamed or raged. I shed some tears but never with real anguish, more with just an overwhelming sense of the wonder of life and that I couldn't bear to lose it.

But Patrick also made me realise that I had perhaps not honestly addressed or sufficiently questioned some of my reactions, especially the possibility of denial. If failing to do that reduces the usefulness of the book, then clearly I must pluck up courage and interrogate myself more rigorously.

How much of my coping strategy had been denial? Was my approach just an act because I needed to be thought positive by other people? How much of this was due to my upbringing, life experience, personality and whatever else makes me who I am? Some of these factors may have contributed both to my positive attitude and to some degree of denial. However tentatively, I will try to explore these issues.

I come from a comfortably privileged family and as children we were expected not only to enjoy our life but also to appreciate how lucky we were. My sisters and I could hardly have been given a happier, more enriching or secure start. Whatever should happen to us later, we could remember that we had already had more than our fair share of good fortune.

And my father set us a fine example. As I said in my tribute at his memorial service:

My father was deeply grateful for his richly varied and long life. He thought he'd had more than his fair share of blessings and happiness. Some might think he also had more than his fair share of sadnesses: the early death of his own mother; the loss of his beloved younger brother, a fighter pilot; the painful years of my mother's long illness and death. Neither his own mother nor his first wife ever knew their grandchildren. Later he had to face the agony of the death of his youngest daughter, Bunny.

Yet he would have instantly dismissed any suggestion that he had had anything but an exceptionally happy life.

Similarly my mother would manage to find good in every experience. No holiday was ever described as anything but exciting, enjoyable and fun even if it had rained every day, the caravan had leaked and one child after another had caught a cold and coughed all night. When something dreadful happened she usually saw it as 'perfectly timed' because it would have been so much worse had it happened the week before.

I could hardly complain about my own lot when I looked at my two sisters. One got cancer at 43 and had the agony of deserting two young children. The other had three episodes of cancer starting in her early fifties and had suffered inestimable distress during her daughter's struggle with manic depression and subsequent death. Cancer at 63, however poor my prognosis, didn't begin to compare. I suppose I could have felt angry that as a family we had been dealt such a treacherous hand. Perhaps it is odd that I didn't. But I didn't.

Anger was not part of my childhood. Both our parents were peace lovers, perhaps to a fault. We were certainly ill prepared for any conflict or aggression we might meet later in life. I don't remember ever hearing my parents have a heated argument. My mother was quite disproportionately distressed by her third child's temper tantrums as a toddler. We were never smacked in anger but only after calculated preparation (which was far worse – and with a hairbrush). Conflict between us three children was strongly, if ineffectually, discouraged.

To say that I never now get angry would be untrue. But it tends to either be a tiresome irritability that is almost entirely deposited, usually unfairly, on Ronald. Or a rather tedious angry stubbornness when something I want is slow to be done. (I am sure those who worked with me must have found this a very unattractive trait.) But these types of anger would have been futile in my recent situation.

Also I did not have the provocation of some patients, of an enduring resentment that a mistake had been made by the doctors, that the diagnosis had been delayed and that my chances of survival were therefore reduced. Ronald suffered from that and still feels angry about it. I had no such problem to cope with.

My family had shown me different ways of handling cancer. I could draw something from my father's stoicism, one sister's acceptance, the other sister's resilience and my husband's humour. Few people could have had a wider or richer choice of role models. Within the family there were also approaches that wouldn't suit me and it was helpful to have seen the downside of these. I would not have wanted secrecy and the mis-understandings and isolation it can cause.

My medical training has also helped me through my diagnosis, treatment and convalescence. As I have already said my professional background and the curiosity that went with it was a huge protection. However negative I might be feeling either from fear, pain or just less than perfect caring, I could nearly always detach myself and look at it as an interesting example of an allergic reaction, a poor doctor/patient relation-ship, an unusual symptomatology, or whatever.

And this protection was greatly reinforced once I had decided to write the book. The worse the experience, the more grist to the story. I would immediately jot down a note or start composing the paragraph concerned in my head, be it in the bath, on the bus or in the clinic waiting room.

Another factor was perhaps my experience of illness and death. Many patients have little previous experience of serious illness, and are disgusted or fearful of its consequences. The word 'cancer' terrifies many – if less so than in the past. I was familiar with disease, with deformity, with patient distress, with surgical operations (and had performed them, however reluctantly, early in my career) and with the realities of dying and death. All this must have made it easier for me.

On occasions I could have been upset, even humiliated, by a response from one or two of the nurses. But again I was protected by the knowledge that I would have wished and demanded the same care for my own patients as I was asking for myself. One nurse clearly resented my request for a painkilling suppository rather than a tablet. I could see a tablet would be nicer for her – and indeed for me – were it not that I knew it would make me vomit. Similarly when I requested an ambulance, rather than sit in a car, for the 75-mile journey home, the scornful reaction of the staff nurse could again have undermined my confidence.

Perhaps, too, the memory of mistakes I had made myself in the past, and insensitivities I had shown, made it easier for me to make allowances for others. For the first time I realised how very difficult it can be for doctors to get it right when talking to patients. Not only do patients vary widely in what they want to hear or not, but any individual patient can change from visit to visit. When my spirits were high I enjoyed the clinic banter and chat about fashion, clothes shopping or the latest film. It made me feel that I was still part of a world wider than the cancer clinic. On other visits I resented any delay at all, any distraction from getting down to the depressing subject of my bowels or my fearsome outlook. Patients often disguise their moods. Doctors are bound sometimes to strike the wrong note.

I had other advantages. Although the doctors were thoughtful in always treating me primarily as a patient, most were conscious that I was also a relatively senior consultant colleague. This may well have led to me being given more time and attention than the average patient, as well as the unexpected perk of an apparently vacant private room.

Most of all I had the 24-hour attention of someone who was prepared to listen and talk about anything – or almost anything – and whenever I wanted. A partner who had himself experienced both cancer and depression. And one who was not only willing but also available, having no obligations to a job, children or any other dependants. He was able to give my needs priority at all times and unselfishly did so. And together we were constantly uplifted by the ever-changing, always beautiful, scenery around us.

I was conscious that this new situation brought bonuses too, many of which I have described in earlier chapters. The most immediate one was relinquishing any caring roles. Throughout my life, chance and circumstance seem frequently to have cast me in that role. Being the eldest child and the only medical member of the immediate family, I often seemed the obvious choice. Carers never feel good enough. It is generally much easier to be the patient.

Finally cheerful patients are easier to like than cranky ones – I knew this from my work. I wanted to keep my friends.

But after all these explanations, was I, as Patrick asked, am I still, in some denial? I don't know. Perhaps that is in itself a sign of denial. Or is it hope? I don't know. Nor do I know where one may merge into the other. Perhaps only others can judge. I am certainly not in denial about the facts in relation to my prognosis: the chances of the cancer returning, of dying quite soon. I am not conscious of fearing a terminal illness and death. Perhaps that is some form of denial as I have never in fact been tested with prolonged severe pain and have no reason to think I would be good at bearing it. I *know* that there is a substantial chance that this may be the last time I see the autumn colours, yet I find that difficult to believe, so I suppose that is denial. Perhaps it doesn't matter. Indeed maybe I should be grateful for it. As Patrick says, denial can help.

Mr Mirza, my surgeon, said that the second year after my operation would be the real test. He is right and I am now, for the first time, scared I won't continue to cope. Different as the circumstances are, I am reminded of a client in our Supertwins Clinic, a mother of triplets who were conceived after IVF treatment. She found the first year much easier than she had expected.

I still remember the vehemence of the letter I received when this mother's babies were six months old. It was at a time when I was vocal in the campaign to discourage infertility specialists from risking giving triplets to their patients. Three babies at the same time, I believed, were neither good for the babies nor their mother – medically or psychologically. The mother wrote to tell me that I was quite wrong. Her babies were flourishing and so was she; she could not be happier with her lot and I should not attempt to deny such pleasures to others.

Eighteen months later this same mother wrote to me again. This time it was a letter of apology. The second year had been shattering. She was exhausted, harassed and depressed. She now wished she could have had her much-loved children one at a time. She ended by encouraging me to continue campaigning.

Whereas many mothers would have been overwhelmed by the practical challenges of three babies, this competent primary school teacher with good family support and adequate financial resources had found the early months straightforward. Much more upsetting were the demands of three two-year-olds and her own frustrations in not being able to give each child the individual attention they needed and deserved and as triplets couldn't possibly have.

Like this mother, the first year for me had not been as hard as I expected. Like her, I knew what I had to do and had the strength and resources to do it. Like her, I could give my full attention to the task on hand. I had little fear of the unknown. I had confidence in my doctors and nurses and in the treatment I was to receive. Unlike many, I had no financial concerns, no pressure to get back to work or to resume domestic duties or childcare. Of course I hated the idea of death but I didn't dwell on it. I was fully occupied doing all I could to avoid it.

But like this mother of triplets the hardest time was yet to come. And as with her, the emotional stress daunted me far more than the physical.

Part Four
The Future

18

BRCA1 Today and Our Family

IN MAY 2006 the Human Fertilisation and Embryology Authority approved pre-implantation genetic diagnosis, or PGD for the BRCA1 and BRCA2 gene mutations, as well as for a gene causing hereditary cancer of the colon (hereditary non-polyposis colorectal cancer or HNPCC).

Pre-implantation diagnosis is a new method for avoiding the transmission of a specific gene from would-be parents to future children. It enables a couple to conceive a child that is biologically their own, yet know that he or she will not be affected by the genetic condition that runs in the family. It uses the now familiar 'test tube' method of in vitro fertilisation where the eggs are retrieved from the woman and the sperm from her partner allowing fertilisation to take place outside the body. One cell is then removed from each of the resulting embryos and tested for the gene defect in question. Only an embryo that is free from the cancer gene would be selected for implantation in the womb.

Previous to the May 2006 decision, approval for PGD had largely been limited to hereditary disorders like cystic fibrosis that would cause lifelong disability or death in infancy or childhood. Using PGD to screen for cancer genes is a controversial move for at least two reasons: not everyone who carries the BRCA1 mutations will necessarily develop cancer (the chance is 80 per cent during a lifetime), and because measures can be taken to both prevent and treat the disease. Moreover the cancer would not develop until much later in life, by which time there may well have been life-changing progress in the prevention, detection and treatment of cancer.

The new ruling from the Human Fertilisation and Embryology Authority allowing PGD for the BRCA1 gene created a dilemma for our family – and no doubt for many others. Following Professor Ponder's advice we had previously agreed that there would be no need to worry the younger family members about our family cancer, until about their late-twenties, unless they themselves raised the subject.

The picture was now quite different. With the possibility of PGD any affected family member could now choose to avoid having a pregnancy which would result in a baby who had inherited our family's cancer gene. Naturally the four nephews and nieces involved could only make decisions about this if they were fully informed well before their first pregnancy. I consulted Bruce Ponder again who agreed that the situation had changed and now we had no option but to speak to the young, all now aged between 18 and 22, before they were likely to be considering pregnancy.

Within our own family the parents differed in their views about the rights and wrongs of PGD. Some felt it was difficult to justify such screening. It was agreed that these differences should be made clear to their children. On the other hand, as all four of them were now adults, in the end they had the right to make the decisions for themselves, so we should not delay in providing them with the necessary information.

Before doing so, we were keen to be prepared for their questions and possible reactions to the information. I was well aware that Felicity's and my own response to the BRCA1 threat had not necessarily been typical. We had never had any doubt that once genetic testing became available, we would be tested, and that meanwhile we wanted to take any reasonable measures to prevent ourselves developing cancer or at least to detect it early. Others may choose to remain in ignorance or, even if tested and found to be a mutation carrier, decide not to take any active measures to avoid cancer.

However I needed to remember that I had myself been slow to see the need for action, let alone to take any active measures, until our immediate family had been hit with Bunny's ovarian cancer. Before that I could well have been accused of being less than conscientious in both my research and action, or simply just in denial.

In the seventies and eighties neither genetic testing nor PGD were yet available. If they had been, would any of the three of us have included PGD and embryo selection in the preventive measures we took? I am glad Ronald and I did not have to make that decision. I do not know what path I would have chosen. Ronald has no doubt. He tells me he would have encouraged me to have PGD but, as he did with our infertility treatment, he would have left the final decision to me. For himself, while seeing the obvious disadvantages of taking the IVF route to pregnancy, he sees no substantial ethical objection to a procedure that can negate an 80 per cent chance of his possible daughters getting breast or ovarian cancer and a 50 per cent chance of his children of either gender transmitting the same curses to his grandchildren. In his view, the choice of a genetically healthy embryo is for him no more interference with nature than, say, postponement of pregnancy – which also produces a different child. In any case he sees much interference as essentially welcome, such as the potentially life-saving treatments of blood transfusion or antibiotics.

Had Bunny still been alive, there might have been differing views between we three sisters. But she wasn't, and it would be particularly hard for Bunny's children, Lizzie and Catherine, that their mother was not there to talk through such complex and sensitive issues.

How and what and when to tell the children about their risk of carrying BRCA1 was discussed among their parents and by Ronald and myself. But we still hadn't come to a conclusion that suited everyone. There was the potential of some of the young being told while others weren't. In the end we were all, in fact, pre-empted by Catherine. She and I were walking among the Gaudi buildings in Barcelona when out of the blue, she asked me about the cancer in our family. What might it mean for her and her sister, Lizzie?

We had always agreed that should the children ask we would answer all their questions truthfully. Within the following few weeks the parents had spoken to the other three. I also wrote a paper that could be given to each of them if appropriate. I thought it might be easier to have the information written down and applicable directly to our own family circumstances rather than have them depend on one of the many general explanations offered on the Internet or in booklets. This is it:

'BRCA1 cancer gene'

For most people who get it, cancer occurs without warning, seemingly out of the blue. However a small proportion of cancers, particularly breast and ovarian cancer, do run in families and are associated with particular genes.

BRCA1, or breast cancer gene, is one of these and runs in the Bryan family. It can be inherited, and passed on, by either male or female members. Children whose mother or father carries the cancer gene will have a 50/50 chance of inheriting the gene themselves.

As this cancer only involves breasts and ovaries it rarely affects men. Nor had there until recently been any way of knowing whether a man had inherited the cancer gene unless one of his daughters developed that kind of cancer.

Your great-grandmother (Grandpa's mother, Silver Bryan) and your great-aunt (Grandpa's sister, Sylvia Wevill) developed cancer of the ovary. So did a number of more distant cousins. However, we did not know whether Grandpa had inherited the cancer gene until Bunny got cancer of the ovary.

Soon after that it became possible to positively identify the BRCA1 cancer gene through a blood test. Felicity and I then arranged to have this blood test and found that we too, like Bunny, were positive.

If a woman has the cancer gene she will not necessarily develop cancer. There is, however, about an 80 per cent chance that she will do so at some stage in life unless she takes action to avoid it. At what age the cancer appears can vary widely. In our family no one has had it before they were 40.

Felicity and I had our ovaries removed once we knew we

didn't want, or couldn't have, any more children. Unfortunately, Felicity later developed breast cancer. Luckily this was caught early and treated. I avoided getting ovarian or breast cancer by having everything at risk removed. Whether the cancer in my pancreas is related to our BRCA1 family gene is not known. It is apparently quite rare.

Some people prefer not to find out whether they have the cancer gene. Clearly such people will not want to have the BRCA1 gene test. Others think it helps to know.

If for example the test proves negative, you can feel reassured and needn't worry any more about it. If you find you do carry the gene, a number of things can be done to prevent any danger of the cancer becoming a serious problem.

Women can have careful and frequent screening of ovaries and breast by ultrasound to detect and treat any cancer as early as possible. Ovaries are more difficult to screen than breasts, so to be (almost) completely safe, ovaries probably need to be removed by your early forties.

As both Felicity and Bunny carried the gene, all four of you have a 50/50 chance of carrying it too. You could all be negative and therefore in the clear. But equally you could all have the bad luck of carrying it. The most likely situation is that some of you will have it and others not.

Until this year there has been no hurry for you even to think about the chances. Even if you were found to be positive there was nothing that needed to be done or even considered until your late-thirties.

The situation has now changed. If you carry the cancer gene, it is now possible to avoid passing it on to any child you may have. A child conceived by someone who carries the cancer gene, either in an egg or a sperm, has a 50/50 chance of inheriting that gene. You all four, therefore, need at least to know about this new option before you think of getting pregnant.

You can avoid having a child with the cancer gene by taking advantage of a new procedure, Pre-implantation Genetic Diagnosis or PGD. This is done using IVF, in vitro fertilisation, or the 'test tube' method. After several eggs have been collected from the woman and fertilised by sperm, the resulting embryos can be tested for the gene. Only an embryo that is negative for the cancer gene would be transferred to the woman's womb.

Many people will not want to even consider PGD but it is important that you at least know what options are available.

Over the next twenty years there are likely to be many improvements in the detection and treatment of cancer and the chance of dying of cancer will certainly decrease. By how much and when, unfortunately no one can say.

All four took the information seriously but without undue alarm. They each talked to me about it at some length when we were holidaying together a few weeks later. Their first reaction was that they would probably go ahead and be tested for the family BRCA1 mutation when practicable. As one was setting off for China the following week and another to Chile, at least two would wait until the following year. They all understood about the option of PGD and embryo selection. Not surprisingly this was a new concept to them and not one about which they wanted to make any immediate decisions. Nor, fortunately, did they need to.

We of the older generation needed to remind ourselves of the importance of confidentiality. The young all know that their parents and I are happy to talk about any concerns they may have and that genetic counsellors are readily available.

But the decisions they are to make are theirs not ours. This applies not only to what they decide and do but also to what they reveal and to whom. It is for them to decide whether they wish to be tested, but also what they choose to say, if anything, about the results or what action, if any, they take after receiving them.

For a family who generally talks openly about personal matters this will require restraint from us. We ought not to enquire about their plans. They have an absolute right, like all adults, to choose how much or little they reveal and to whom. And we have no right to expect or request more.

19

Preparing for Death and Life

A FEW DAYS before she died a friend described her situation as like waiting for a train and not knowing when it would come. I understand that feeling except I am still hoping that my train will be cancelled.

In August 2006 we spent a week in the small mountain town of Bagnone in Liguria. Our B & B was in an old mansion house next to the church and we were woken each morning to the sound of its bells. I welcomed this until the last day, 10 August. Had it now become a death knell? It was six months to the day since I had finished my chemotherapy. From now on I must be prepared for the cancer to return. Ronald and I went into the church, lit a candle and prayed.

During my chemotherapy, and for the six months that followed, I had felt safe. I had been told that my cancer would not recur during that time. Nearly 40 years as a doctor had repeatedly taught me that medicine is not an accurate science, and never less accurate than when predicting the outlook for a cancer patient. Nevertheless 10 August had become a crucial date in my diary.

From that date, life was to become much harder.

By October 2006, 15 months after my surgery, I am out-wardly back to 'normal'. I am my old self with a new figure. I look very well and everyone keeps telling me so. I need more rest than I used to and my bowels remain a bit of a problem. They are uncomfortable and sometimes painful and erratic. I have to be more cautious with my diet but on the whole none of this stops me doing what I want to do or causes me undue embarrassment.

Inwardly, I am far from normal. I am thrashing about, bewildered. The swinging moods of the past have returned. During the downs I find life difficult. Unless I am to live in denial, I must face two scenarios – of death and of survival – and being the planner I am, must prepare for both. And meanwhile I must live both. Live well but inevitably in the shadow of death.

With a cancer there is really only one question: is it going to kill me? In some ways even a serious cancer is easier than many illnesses. There is little one can do to prevent it recurring so there are no tiresome precautions to take. You are often well until you are 'dying'. It is not like someone with heart or lung problems who may be unwell for many years and who knows that if they are not careful, they may well accelerate their death. And, however careful they are, they may still die without warning.

Those of us who have had cancer have often got rid of the offending organ or at least the part with the tumour and there may then be no reason why we shouldn't live on as long as anyone else and in good health. Or at least until the cancer returns. Of course some of us will have tiresome side effects from our surgery, like me with my bowels and Ronald with his swollen leg. But these are trivial compared with the continuous pain, disability, deformity or daily apprehensions that can occur with many other diseases.

Nevertheless, however well you are today, cancer brings uncertainty. It might come back next week, next month, next year. No one can tell me. Previous success in life serves you badly when it comes to coping with something that can't be changed, like infertility or death. I have usually tackled difficult things with determination, and within my modest ambitions I have usually succeeded. Now no matter how hard I try, 'success' is not in my hands. Indeed 'success' may need to be redefined. Success may not be measured by how long I live but how well I die.

I hate uncertainty but certainty for me could only mean death. Statistical survival rates are crucial numbers for cancer patients but where will I be in them? In what percentile? I hate not knowing. I want to know now. Should I prepare to live or prepare to die? It seems no one can tell me. In one way dying could be easier than living. It would be less complicated and, as I have said, I do not dread the process. I just can't bear the thought of not living. So I must face the two scenarios.

First, the dying scenario. What about the last stages of my terminal illness? From the practical viewpoint I don't worry about this. We designed our house so that we could stay here to the end of our lives, and, when the time comes, die here. Our bedroom, bathroom and studies are downstairs. We have room for a live-in carer. I dream of dying in our own bed with only the birds and their hanging feeders between me and the Black Mountains.

Uncontrollable pain is sometimes the reason for a terminally ill patient to be moved from home. Our GP lives a short way up the hill and the practice has an excellent team of community nurses. I am confident that, with support from the local hospice, they would control my pain.

The only other reason for leaving home would be for Ronald's well-being. However well he is supported, my 24-hour presence through a prolonged illness could be an intolerable emotional strain. Certainly if I became confused or just plain awkward. We have no children to share this burden or help him decide whether I ought to be moved. So, well in advance, I shall ask one or two very close friends to help him make that decision, if and when the time comes, regardless of, or only slightly regarding, my protestations.

Psychologically and emotionally, I don't think I worry about dying or death. I just don't want to waste a moment of the last and biggest experience that I shall ever have. I have seen more happiness given and received in the last days of someone's life than at any other time. But I have also seen a lot of unhappiness, some of it avoidable. If Ronald is with me, my pain is under control and together we have received Holy Communion, my only remaining concern would be for anyone with whom I had 'unfinished business' or unresolved misunderstandings. I hope there won't be any. I have no excuse. I have been given time enough to face them.

As I have said before, it is difficult for most people to know who they will want with them as they die, or indeed in the final hours. A few choose to be alone. Many fear being alone and are comforted by the presence of someone close. I don't think I *fear* being alone, just the shortage of friends that that isolation might represent. I know that Ronald and I would want to be together. But he couldn't be there for 24 hours a day for what might be many days of waiting. Of course I can't know how I would feel when the time came but I do know I should hate anyone to be uncomfortable or to feel that they had to be with me.

For some people to be with a friend as that person dies may be a joy and privilege as it was for me with both Bunny and my father. But just as in life some people like to say goodbye through the car window as they drop their friend at the station while others are still waving on the platform long after the friend has settled down with novel and sandwiches, so with death. I am sure that some of my closest friends would prefer to say goodbye well ahead of my departure. Others may come to the station, some may sit with me on the platform, even help me on to the train but only a very few will want to wait for the guard's whistle. And anyway Ronald might not be in the mood to host a large farewell party.

Whatever happens I hope and trust that Ronald would not delay the guard. We have both seen dying friends whose pain of parting has been unwittingly increased by partners who couldn't bear to let their loved one go, who tried desperately to hold them back against their wish and inclination. Like Bunny during her last week, who said that 'now that the time has come, I feel an impatience', many people who have striven valiantly for many months to live, know when the time has come to die. There is no greater gift than to release a dear friend or partner to do so in peace and dignity, surrounded by love.

Who would be with me in those final days would depend not only on our mutual comfort but who is available. Dying can rarely be conveniently timed. I have no doubt that there are a number of relations and friends who would be prepared to come if I asked them. But I hope that only those who really wanted to come would accept the invitation.

Clearly if I die, it is easy for me. I shall have no price to pay, no persisting worries. What of others – will any suffer? Thanks to our wide circle of friends quite a number of people would miss me but so they would if I emigrated to Australia, and the small gap I left would be quickly filled. For a few in whose lives I have a unique place and they in mine, there would be a true and perhaps irreplaceable loss. That is the price of love. But memories would live on and continue to enrich their lives just as memories of other family and friends who have died have continued to enrich mine.

Ronald is the only one who would find a physical gap in his life. His pattern of life would certainly change. We had always assumed our deaths would be separated by some years. Now they may not happen in the order we expected. At the start I was deeply concerned as to how he would manage. Now I know he can manage on his own, perhaps better than I would. He would find life more peaceful and more orderly without me. But he would miss me a lot and I find that part of the scenario too painful to grapple with yet.

We have yet to talk in any detail as to what would happen to him after I died. Big decisions as to how and where he would choose to live are yet to be discussed. He loves Quercwm, the Golden Valley, the people and our garden. However practical it may be to move into a smaller place I would be surprised if he didn't want to stay. He would clearly be able to live at Quercwm longer if there was someone to help him, particularly with the garden and driving. But Ronald values his peace and any lodger would need to be independent.

Fortunately our house was designed with a bedroom that could become self-contained with its own kitchenette. But it still needed its own bathroom. So, despite Ronald's protests, a shower room has now been installed. I was determined that I should be here to see this through. Until finished, Ronald continued to think it one of my least good ideas – which often involve mess.

Although I can never hope to emulate the orderliness of my father, at least I would like to leave my affairs in some sort of order so that Ronald doesn't have a depressing mountain of muddle to sort out, or that he has to make emotionally testing arrangements. For most of us, preparing for death is not only a new experience but different from any other preparation. Usually you prepare while looking forward to the objective event. The only reason for postponement is unreadiness. For death I should like to be fully prepared then forget the funeral arrangements and the will and enjoy as long as possible all the things that I won't be able to take with me.

I am lucky. I am unlikely to be taken by surprise. If my cancer returns, my terminal illness is likely to last several months, or at least some weeks. Meanwhile I live in limbo and must learn to do so with more equanimity. Otherwise these precious months, weeks or days will be wasted.

So, to the second scenario: survival and the challenges that it poses. Why is it that the thought of living on can be so daunting? Why is life so much harder now than last year, so much harder than I had expected? It isn't only the uncertainty. Kate Carr, writing about her own experience after gruelling treatment for cancer, helped me in my struggle to understand:

The reason why it is hard to survive – and to write about surviving is because everyone, including me, knows it could be worse. I am so lucky to survive – I should be leaping out of bed every morning, jumping for joy! How selfish and self-indulgent when many are so much worse off and dying.[9]

The difficulty is trying to get back to a normal life while abandoning the curious security of being an invalid, one whose world is protected, safe within its own limits, insulated from the stresses and strains of ordinary life and exposed only to the loving concern of friends. Now I must face these normal stresses again and all the irritations and frustrations that go with broken dishwashers, tax accounts that won't add up, long waits on the telephone to change an eye appointment, the lost key.

I had been looking forward to relinquishing the recipient role. For a year friends had been wonderfully generous with their attention and care. Now it is my turn to think about them but I am finding it hard. Moreover I must often confuse people by apparently wanting them to regard me as recovered, but then constantly talking about myself and my cancer.

At a party recently a kind man, who I had only met once before, asked me what I was doing these days. Fifteen minutes later he was still sympathetically listening to the details of my illness. I keep resolving to talk about more interesting subjects – but the awful truth is that at present I find nothing more gripping than my cancer. It has become an almost total preoccupation.

Yet there is also nothing more important to me than my friends. And I fear I shall lose many if I go on like this. I pray I won't.

[9] Carr, Kate, *It's Not Like That Actually*, Vermilion, London, 2004

I wish I could be more like my sister-in-law, Anthea, who, whatever her pains and worries, always replies 'I'm fine thanks'. We have sometimes wanted a more candid answer, but now I really admire her self-restraint.

The constant reminders of my cancer don't help. First my scars: my botched appendicectomy and various cuts and burns are just records or relics of the past, of my history, not my present. But the two inelegant mastectomies and the large beautifully healed abdominal scar are different. They are reminders of ongoing vulnerability.

The trials of late-middle age, a stiff neck in the morning, backache after gardening, creaking knees, headaches after red wine, were all well established before my cancer. But now each twinge could represent cancer spreading in the bowel, to the bone, to the brain. And more unsettling than anything else is the weird orchestral activity in my insides. Perhaps the fears are even greater for those of us with medical backgrounds. Medical knowledge combined with only a little hypochondria can quickly turn a minor symptom into a convincing lethal disease.

However long I last, I may not be able to relinquish fears of the cancer recurring. I am not alone. Last week I met a healthy-looking friend who had been free from any signs or symptoms of bowel cancer since her operation 10 years ago. She confessed she still lives with a daily fear of it recurring. In truth, her chance of dying from a spread from her bowel cancer to another part of her body is probably now much less than from some other cause.

As I come towards the end of the book, I increasingly feel I am making an awful lot of fuss about only one person. Not exactly making a meal of it, or a mountain of a molehill – but just forgetting how tiny my problems are in the great scheme of things. After all, over 15,000 young children are dying every day from malnutrition. And the terrorist attacks on the London Underground in July 2005 suddenly killed 52 people only a few days before my operation. In practical terms, at least, most of those who died were needed much more than I am. They were younger, had more dependants, were still working and had more to offer for the future. I do not even have my own children to worry about. Even at a personal level, since my cancer started, two friends have been diagnosed with pancreatic cancer. One has already died, the other is unlikely to survive more than a few months. A colleague has just dropped dead from a heart attack leaving 12-year-old twin daughters. What am I fussing about? I should be rejoicing to be alive and as well as I am. I *want* to rejoice.

World tragedies may more easily be seen in perspective, however awesome, than particular personal tragedies. We must each struggle our own way through our own difficulties, anxieties and tragedies. I know this from years of work with bereaved parents. Parents often compare their own losses with those of others and sometimes feel they must defend their own loss as if it was not fully appreciated. Mothers who had lost their only baby sometimes made those who had lost a twin but still had a surviving baby, feel guilty about their grief. Those who had lost an older child were sometimes not sensitive to the loss of a baby and even less of one before it was born.

Losses cannot be compared or slotted into a hierarchy. We each can only try honestly to recognise and acknowledge how we feel. That is how it is for each of us – neither better nor worse than other people's experience. Comparing losses is unhelpful and pointless and can be cruel. I have not written about my own fears and losses to suggest that my experience is universal or transferable and certainly not to suggest that it is uniquely difficult. I have done it in the hope it may help someone to usefully reflect on his or her own experiences, fears, irrationalities and uncertainties.

Meanwhile I am struggling to re-establish my identity and role. Who am I now? For over 30 years I was a paediatrician and a specialist in twins and triplets. Last year I was a cancer sufferer, an invalid. Now I am no longer an invalid nor am I an interesting case at the hospital. This year's seriously ill patients have replaced me. I cannot any more share the camaraderie of the Cancer Clinic. I am warmly greeted on my three-monthly visits but I have lost touch with the week-by-week lives of staff and patients in the chemotherapy room. I am no longer foremost in the thoughts of the GP, the vicar or our other neighbours. Rightly there are others who deserve their attention much more.

Even for Ronald, the relief of having me still here may be beginning to wear off. We are back to the usual MTs of any partnership. Nothing serious, nothing dramatic. Far less serious, so far at least, than many. A *Guardian* article had it that 25 per cent of marriages broke up in the first year of cancer and another 12 per cent were threatened.[10] Much of the time I mind the MTs no more than I ever did. But then I suddenly get overwhelmed and fly at him. 'How can we waste time arguing whether glasses do or don't go in the dishwasher?' I might rail at him. 'How can you fuss about global warming when I leave the

[10] *Guardian*, 8 April 2006

odd light on – when life should be treasured – and we may not have long of it?' These emotional outbursts are hard on Ronald, especially since they are so unpredictable. And when he knows how upset I would be if he exploded in the same way.

Because our time together may be so limited I am perhaps unfairly resentful when we spend time on what I consider rather superfluous activities like vegetable growing. When I (fairly) gently enquired whether we really needed 64 tomato plants as he was now the only one able to eat their fruit, he sighed as he replied that perhaps it was a sign of his denial of my illness.

Of course, in many ways I should be grateful. I have been given an unusual opportunity to rethink my life, to review the past, to plan the future. Within my physical and financial limits I can do it in whatever way Ronald and I together would like. And I have had plenty of time to reflect on the possibilities. But still I want and need more peaceful time. Time that is not cluttered with the turmoil of uncertainty. Once this book is finished, time just 'to be' is something to which I most look forward.

It is 11 November 2006. I had intended to end my story yesterday, exactly nine months after I finished my chemotherapy and three months after the bell tolled in Bagnone. But today, Armistice Day will, I hope, be a turning point for me. A friend with whom I had not spoken for about six months or so rang on a business matter. Towards the end of our conversation she enquired how I was. Yet again, it all poured out.

She responded with the authority of the head teacher she is and of somebody who had been through a serious cancer experience herself. Ten years ago the chances of her surviving the year were small. She knew those times of despair and confusion and the horrors of uncertainty. She said it was only when she resolved to be in that tiny percentage who survived her particular cancer that she could get on positively with her life. 'Of course,' she said, 'you may not survive but you must believe you will.'

Epilogue

SPRING CAME EARLY to Quercwm in 2007. Outside our window a noisy trio of magpies woke us up each morning and the apple trees were in precocious bloom. Far away across the valley Hay Bluff was greening. It felt good to be alive and here.

Although I was not back to the energy I'd had in the Cevennes (limplustre was a new word a friend coined), I was stable and there was enough in the tank to travel with Ronald round South Africa's Cape Province in January to meet far-flung members of my family and continue the detective hunt into our genes, and then in February to go to Chile to visit my niece, Catherine, who was doing her gap year in a school in the foothills of the Andes.

At times I truly believed that train would not come after all.

But only two weeks after my return from Chile in February I heard it rumble towards me again. It was during a jolly weekend with a group of friends in Shropshire.

The food was delicious, the talk invigorating, but during a 20-minute walk after lunch, I ached all over and felt I might run out of energy before we got back. Lying in bed that night, I began to prepare myself for more bad news.

Epilogue

A few weeks later, I had a scan and blood tests at the Birmingham Hospital, which, to my surprise, were perfectly normal. I should have been relieved; I was not.

It was suggested then that my symptoms – loss of energy, aches and pains – might be due to a deficiency in my diet, no surprise after major abdominal surgery. I was happy to clutch at this straw. There were plenty of diversions during this time: the Hay Festival of Literature, visits from friends. At the beginning of June, I went to the triennial International Congress for Twin Studies in the lovely Gothic city of Ghent where I had a wonderful welcome from friends from all over the world, many of whom I only saw on these occasions. But underneath I felt the now familiar dread that this might be the last time we would be together and the sadness of not being able to say this and say goodbye.

A lovely summer followed at Quercwm. Expeditions into Wales, parties, picnics with friends, lessons in yoga and singing; suppers out on the terrace where, quietly tired, we watched the sun set over the mountains and new dawns with the garden bursting with flowers.

It was life with one battery missing – leaving lunches early for naps in the afternoon; theatre with friends but no energy for supper afterwards. But it was a good life nevertheless, and we savoured every moment, with our minds on the poor survival statistics.

But when the new crop of raspberries came in, I began to wonder if I was picking them for the last time. The nutritional tests now showed that I was very depleted in minerals and certain enzymes, and so I began a daunting daily regime of swallowing 16 tablets of minerals, enzymes and vitamins. Even at the best of times, I'm not a good swallower but I was still clinging to the nutritional straw of hope.

In July, still feeling limplustre but with no definite diagnosis, Ronald and I went away again to the Champernowne Trust's summer course, near Brecon, where I had so enjoyed the swimming, the dancing and the singing the year before. No swimming this year – the sky was grey throughout, the river Usk tumultuous, fast flowing and dangerous. The weather had changed and so had I. The year before I had been celebrating. This year I was unhappy and oddly hungry for the news I dreaded.

Things were changing day by day and, looking back, I can see what a strange time this was, dangling between thoughts of death and tantalised by glimpses of an exciting new literary life opening up around the corner. For my book, this book that had been my lifeline and sometimes my refuge, was suddenly out in the shops and had been given a thrilling reception. It was serialised in the *Daily Mail* and featured in *The Times*. There were interviews, radio programmes, enthusiastic letters from doctors and counsellors, a rave review in the *Lancet*, invitations to lecture in the States, Australia and at home.

The professional recognition from the medical journals was unexpected and deeply satisfying, but just as pleasing were letters from readers. One told me that reading the book had been such a liberating experience it had made her laugh – and cry – out loud.

'Cancer,' she explained, 'is something that has always weighed heavily on me – since my mother had breast cancer when I was 14. It was a very traumatic time. She had a mastectomy and that was it. Cancer over, nothing to talk about

– and still to this day we don't really talk about it. I never saw her scar or talked about death. Good stiff-upper-lip stuff. I have always been convinced I would get it and endlessly worry about lumps and pains. Since reading your book, a huge cloud has lifted. I have finally realised that you don't just die or recover, but you can continue to live and fully appreciate life – and not just curl up in abject terror.'

Hearing that meant so very much to me. It alone justified writing the book.

Praise, of course, is always wonderfully sustaining, and the sense that my suffering had helped others kept me going for months. Yet the haunting sense that all was not well persisted. I could hear that train again.

It is now August 2007. I am sitting, heart thumping, in the Cancer Clinic at Birmingham Hospital once more. My friend Julia is with me. On the other side of the desk is Dr Daniel Palmer, a young consultant oncologist. He is quietly, compassionately, confirming all my worst fears. The cancer markers in my blood are raised. The CT scan shows signs that the tumour has returned. Doctor Palmer, probably young enough to be my son, shows courage as well as kindness. He looks me in the eye, unflinching, tells me there is no likelihood of an actual cure, says I might lead a worthwhile life for some months. There is a feeling of mutual respect.

The train is suddenly screaming down the track, but how complex we humans are. Once again I feel relief at the uncertainty being over. A kind of calm descends on me as we discuss the list of diminishing options available to me – chemotherapy is one of them because there has been a gap since my last treatment. I even joke with Julia that professional pride has been salvaged too – *I told them I was ill!* It is not until we get outside, that we hug each other and cry.

I can so easily understand people who at this point decide to go home and fade away gracefully. But, for me, the decision to carry on with any treatment available was instant. To my surprise, I had a new career – the exploration of familial cancers – and this provided new stimulation in life and new sources of strength. I had no doubt that every day was precious and I wanted to go for every one available.

I was all set to start a second round of chemotherapy on 21 September 2007. Before that I was scheduled to make my tour to the north of England that would complete the launch of my book. This included giving a lecture in York at the annual conference of the British Society of Geneticists, another lecture at the Centre for Life in Newcastle, where I would be introduced by my old friend Professor John Burn. Later I was to address the annual general meeting of Homestart, Leicester, where the theme of my lecture was 'Grasping Opportunities'.

Then, on 26 August, two astonishing email messages came within 24 hours.

The first was from a geneticist friend, Dr Georgia Trench, in Brisbane, the second from John Burn. Both asked me if I had heard of this brand new treatment that was specific to BRCA1 cancers and which was having exciting results in preliminary tests.

Neither of my friends minced their words: the treatment, only available at the Royal Marsden Hospital in Sutton, Surrey, would be arduous – a weekly 320-mile round trip from Quercwm. And it would be tough, each time involving a day of blood tests and scans. I would be given daily tablets of Kudos, as well as a monthly chemotherapy infusion. Either might produce unwelcome side effects, including the possibility of hair loss which I'd dreaded so much in the early days. The treatment would also be unpredictable – it had previously only been tried on people with BRCA1 breast and ovarian cancer. I later learned that I, together with one other, would be the first patient with pancreatic cancer to enter the trial.

What is interesting to me now is that my immediate response was not one of excitement or enthusiasm. In fact I was quite exhausted by this new prospect. I knew that the original chemotherapy plan would in fact only delay the inevitable but suddenly I found the thought of another treatment – even if it did save me – quite overwhelming. I felt I did not have the energy for it.

But by the morning, my attitude had changed. It was not just that this was a possible lifeline. I realised that as a doctor I felt some obligation to help advance this trial. And after all I was about to give a lecture entitled, 'Grasping Opportunities'.

Wednesday 12 September 2007 was a bumper day! Highlighted in my diary for many months, I'd planned a party at the Royal Society of Medicine in Wimpole Street to thank my friends, to mark the launch of the book and to celebrate, somewhat belatedly, my sixty-fifth birthday. Ronald was master of ceremonies and over 200 people were expected – there were godchildren who hadn't seen each other since our wedding, 29 years ago; friends from my Yorkshire childhood and medical school; colleagues from the twin world. Patrick Pietroni was to give a speech, also my publisher Clare Hulton from Vermilion.

Such a surreal day. On the morning of the party, when I might have been at the hairdressers, I was being driven by my friend and colleague, Faith Hallett, down to the Royal Marsden.

I am used to being inside hospitals, having spent decades in them. But when you are there to look down the barrel of a gun, the view changes. The next three hours were spent in preliminary discussions with the research team about the trial and whether I was a suitable case for treatment. It was made clear to me that their final decision would depend upon scans and further tests. A few moments later, I was sitting in a cubicle in my hospital gown waiting for the nurse to take the first blood test of the day. I felt stripped bare and yet hopeful; I so wanted this treatment to work.

By six that evening, and back in Central London, I was putting on my glad rags – a glamorous black dress sequinned with butterflies. My sister Felicity had given it to me. It felt most unlike me and I loved wearing it. While I was getting dressed, I anxiously rehearsed my speech, worrying whether I would have the stamina I'd need for this long evening. I'd invested enormous emotional energy in it – a reunion with lots of friends and colleagues I hadn't seen for many years.

Once I was at the party, I loved every moment of it. Waves of family, then friends, arrived until the great glazed atrium was full. After the speeches, our friends from the Champernowne Trust lustily led the guests in the three verses of 'Singing the Life'. I felt a surge of satisfaction, qualified only by the inevitable sadness of the second verse which goes: 'I sing the death in store for all of us…' I knew in my heart that I would probably not see many of these dear and loyal friends again. But, on the other hand, was I in danger of having more last appearances than

Dame Nelly Melba? If you've said you are going, shouldn't you just go?

That night, exhausted by the party, and yet thrilled by it all, I lay in bed and thought about the last few months: the best and the worst of times.

Injections, late-night fears, frustration at feeling so feeble, the difficulties and pleasures of writing this book – the sense that the spirit could go on working if only it could find a way. The joy of sitting with Ronald in the garden and feeling as well as seeing, even more vividly than before, the beauty of trees, and birds, and skies.

Having a project, a task, a job to perform during these past two years had been so important for me. Bunny had always felt the same, not wanting to be seen as a set of symptoms. And it gives you other things to talk about when people come to see you. Everyone finds their own way in this, of course. Some, if they are well enough, travel. One young mother I knew made a recipe book for her children. But for me, writing it all down made me feel like the real me.

But I must not wax too lyrical. Dying has also been harder than I expected; much harder at times.

When I thought about dying before my cancer was diagnosed, I imagined I might have become a more peaceful, philosophical and submissive version of myself as I went gentle into that good night. It never occurred to me that life would carry on being so tantalisingly interesting, that even at death's door there might be new goals, treats to look forward to. In short, that I would want so much to go on living.

It was now late autumn; the trees were shedding their leaves, the rabbits still proliferating. After all the excitement of the book's publication launch and the tour of the North had died down, I was tired, and I knew I had to give my whole attention to gathering my strength for the rigorous treatment that lay only two weeks ahead. One of the hardest lessons learned at this time was how to ask for help from friends without feeling I was putting them out.

Sometimes, I was ruefully reminded of a wonderful remark made to me by a woman aged 104: 'When you are old, never apologise for being a nuisance. You *are* a nuisance.'

But could I really ask busy friends to drive me to London all the way from the Welsh Marches. Would this be a bridge too far? I worried that I might be sick during these journeys, or be caught short and have to stop; or that they would feel obliged to drive me when it was inconvenient.

In the end Judy Gowing, who had once organised conferences with me at the Hammersmith Hospital, took the problem out of my hands. She drew up a roster of friends happy to take turns driving me to each hospital visit. I am so glad she did. I've always thought that the car was a great place in which to talk to friends and with each one of my drivers there was openness, a freedom about our conversations that I will always treasure. We laughed, we cried, we shared cups of coffee and chocolate muffins at motorway service stations. I told them about my fears for myself and for Ronald. They often told me about the death or illness of a parent or a loved friend. In short we revealed things we might have felt for years but which British reserve, or lack of time, had stopped us saying. So lesson learned: don't be frightened of asking for help. People like helping. And if you love someone, tell them.

Having friends with me also helped me not get too nervous

about what lay ahead. Although, as I had already experienced in Birmingham, good specialist units exude reassurance and competence, this was still an emotional roller coaster for me. But once again at the Marsden I was impressed with how cutting-edge science could be combined with compassion.

One nurse talked to me for a good hour about my pain control, to make sure she had all the exact details. The charming African food orderly questioned me with wonderful precision about what I would like to eat. I know the National Health is not famous for fine dining, but I was astonished at the quality they produced.

After various blood tests showed my cancer markers were raised, a CT scan showed the cancer had returned but in the form of scattered nodes rather than one large mass. It may seem strange to relate, but once I knew the cancer had returned and I'd be accepted on the trial, I felt very positive, excited and interested. The doctor part of me was intrigued by the process, and by how the medical staff went about their work. But, at the same time, the vulnerable patient in me knew I was reaching the end of my possible lifelines. I had to believe in it, and I did. It was a split screen reality. When my first treatment was over and I returned home, I revised and signed my will, did my income tax, tidied the attic.

We kept up the treats, not always wholly successfully. We went to London for *Aida* at the Coliseum, but I felt groggy and Ronald's gammy leg kept falling off his stool, so we left in the first interval, giggling like naughty children as we ate ice cream on our tube journey home to our friends. But the following weekend, we went to stay most happily with friends in Dorset, and to a magical candle-lit performance of Mozart's *Great Mass in C Minor* in Christchurch Abbey. And that is another thing I would say: keep the treats going right up until the very end, if at all possible.

There was a crisis during this time, which frightened me. The course of the treatment was complicated. At one stage my bowels became partly blocked, the pressure built up and I was unable to eat any solids at all. My weight which had remained steady at eight and a half stone for the two and a half years since diagnosis, now started to drop dramatically. At the beginning of November I was losing a pound a day and did so for 10 days.

I became very weak and was admitted to the Marsden's palliative care ward. The staff were again impressively gentle and efficient. I felt greatly reassured to realise that this support would be available to me here or in a hospice. I was hugely relieved when they managed to sort out this mechanical problem, for I so longed to continue with my treatment, even though I knew I couldn't expect any definite results for some time.

But it was a false dawn.

At the end of November, after six weeks of treatment, I drove to London with a friend, feeling almost elated. My appetite was back – we celebrated by eating half an almond slice at a petrol station. I was going full steam ahead with the treatment that might save me. That night, undressing for bed at the Marsden, I said a silent prayer that the treatment could be continued. The following day, sitting behind floral curtains, waiting for the doctor to arrive, I was still feeling remarkably optimistic. I had a scan, and at 10.30 in the morning in a bright sunlit room, the specialist told me, in a broken voice, that the treatment has failed. The tumour has become larger, the cancer markers are up, there is no indication of benefit and there could be harm. The treatment must therefore be stopped. At once.

My thoughts were in a turmoil: huge disappointment, shock, fear and also sorrow for the doctors who had so wanted my treatment to work.

To add to the confusion, I was due to speak about my book at the Hay Winter Literary Festival, only three days later. I was to give a short talk and be interviewed by Julian Mitchell, the playwright. I decided not to tell my audience of this sudden reverse. I felt that the sad news would get in the way of my more positive messages. But could I cope? Ronald and Felicity assured me that they could fill the gap somehow, if it got too much for me. Even so, that day began as an ordeal. I put on my pink silk dress but I felt quite sick and unsure whether I could go through with it. I was glad in the end that I hadn't cancelled. I didn't fall over and my answers to necessarily tough questions from Julian were well received. Afterwards I felt a really sustaining tide of love and support from the audience. But, of course, there is a price: I felt very drained and slept for several hours.

The following day, Ronald and I sent out an email sharing our bad news.

Quercwm Update.

Very dear friends,

As many of you know, I have been having some new experimental treatment at the Royal Marsden Hospital for the recent recurrence of my pancreatic cancer.

Last week I had the disappointing news that this treatment has not only failed to stop the cancer but is having side effects that could themselves be dangerous. Meanwhile, a scan has shown that the cancer is definitely progressing.

I have therefore now been taken off all treatment except painkillers for a fortnight. Should this rest strengthen me sufficiently, there may be a chance to try some other treatment. But I am told this is unlikely and that I may now have only a few months to live. Most of the time I find this hard to believe and continue to enjoy and treasure each day. The pain is largely controlled and we are still planning some treats (including three days on the Rhine later this week!) And also, I hope, some more writing and even lecturing. But I also want to be prepared so must sadly accept that there are some dear friends who I may not see again. Or even be able to talk, or write to, as much as I should have liked.

We expect to stay most of the time peacefully at Quercwm where we have wonderful support from friends and neighbours and our family doctor living next door. Emails are usually our best forms of contact. We prefer to avoid telephone calls between 1 and 3.30pm and after 8pm. Ronald will continue to send an occasional report. Meanwhile we shall know you are continuing to hold us in your hearts. For that we are more grateful than we shall ever be able to say. You have already helped to give us two of our happiest years.

With our fondest love to you all
Libby/Elizabeth with Ronald

PS: Please feel free to forward this email to anyone who you think would like to know what is happening to us.

Epilogue

So, the light has changed again, and my greatest challenge now is to face up to 'Dying the death that is there for all of us'. At times I have had the strangest, most unexpected, feelings of excitement about it. When I tried to explain this to a friend recently, I said it was like being offered an exotic and perhaps dangerous world tour when you'd rather muck about at home with your friends.

The sublime and the mundane are mixed. I still get ridiculously anxious about small things: untidy cupboards; will Ronald remember to cancel the milk or phone the dentist. But maybe such anxieties mask the gathering sorrow of parting from loved ones and of leaving this life, which I have loved so very much, in so many ways.

Shopping at Sainsbury's – don't laugh – was another intense experience recently. It was our first trip for quite a while and I saw everything with fresh eyes. It was disturbing, as if I wasn't part of the world, and didn't want to be in the world.

Yet I am still gasping at the beauty of things: at Hay Bluff this week coated in snow and with the purest blue sky above it; at the thrush who sits framed by leaves and jewel-like berries on the bird table outside our bedroom window.

I am longing to write my next book. I am cross that my sister Felicity will now wear my new padded coat from Land's End, yet pleased she took it with such alacrity.

My mind is going back more often to my childhood: I see Felicity – who comes to stay with me every weekend now – galloping her little pony down the track through the woods. Such a little thing, and so fearless. I see my mother, the beach at Whitby. I remember the camps on the Yorkshire Moors for my many godchildren. One of the shyest of the children recently wrote pages to me to say how much they'd meant to her.

Singing the Life

I know my days are numbered now, and I still can't quite believe it. There is still so much to look forward to. It is the middle of January, my weight has fallen to six and a half stone. My GP and two district nurses come to see me every day now to help me adjust the morphine dose and flow and help with any other worries. Too much and I could become confused and certainly tend towards over-anxiety.

My nephew Max comes back from China especially to spend time with me. We decide to combine his visit with a harp concert.

Ten come for lunch, family members and close friends. 'Matron' Ronald prepares a delicious meal of smoked salmon, smoked guinea fowl, mixed salads, followed by poached pears and apple ginger ice cream.

I am too weak to get up for lunch, but my nephews and nieces take turns to join me in my bedroom at different points of the meal. I wanted to see each on their own, and this time is very precious to me. It takes the wisdom of 19-year-old Catherine to tell me that quality of life is what matters now, not the number of my days.

After lunch, I lie on the sofa surrounded by family and a few close friends. And a harpist, Catrin, a beautiful woman pregnant with her third child who I know from Champernowne days, who sits in the corner of the room, bathed in golden light. Ronald reads the Sanskrit poem that I love so much: 'Look to this day, for it is life, the very best of life.'

The harpist plays the Bach Partita she has agreed to play at my funeral. My dear friend, Frances Hancock, who will soon be conducting it, reads Wordsworth's hymn of praise to the countryside, 'Lines composed overlooking Tintern Abbey', and I am struck again by the simple truth of his words about those 'little nameless, unremembered acts of kindness and of love' that are 'the best portion of a good man's life'.

There have been so many examples of these in the last few months. The 3am emails from friends sending their love, the birdseed and a fruitcake left at the front door, the friend who came to help me tidy the attic, unexpected deliveries of chicken soup.

All these people mean so much to me. Some are crying now and some are smiling. They've come to be with me.

There is, contained within this darkening room, an over-whelming sense of the sorrow and beauty of life. I look at the fire, at Ronald sitting in his chair. He must be tired after preparing lunch, but he is smiling at me, he holds my hand. Felicity sits close to me with her back to the window. Beyond her three or four dark birds are flying in formation and then melting into the mist forming over Hay Bluff. The whole day feels for me like one of those openings in life when you see into the heart of things. Like a kind of funeral, but better, because I was there.

A Husband's
Afterword

FOLLOWING OUR AFTERNOON with the harp, Libby had just a month in which to say her last goodbyes. She had shrunk to just six stones, but was still smiling. After she had turned down the last treatment offered to her she had gained a special sort of peace and spent hours on the couch by the sitting room window drinking in the valley's loveliness.

She was heart-rendingly frail but the automatic morphine curbed most of the pain and, in sudden bursts of energy, she went through cupboards and sorted piles of stuff – clothes, shoes, jewellery, books, toys – for family, friends and Oxfam. Each evening I trundled the old invalid chair next to the Aga where for much of the night she answered emails, made soup or ice cream and wrote out my chores for the next day, and for when she had died. Then she would sleep till seven in the morning, late for her. We knew she was on borrowed time but she devoured each day hungrily. The district nurses were amazed that anyone on so much morphine could still potter about.

Each setback seemed to be quickly followed by refreshed delight: a niece's phone call, a generous letter, a good review of her book, a (wonderfully unrealistic) invitation to speak in

Brisbane or Chicago. Three times a television team interviewed her about first and last things and how best to die. For half an hour she would blossom, speaking as lucidly as ever, before subsiding on the pillows. But while I admired her fortitude and bravery, I was steadily growing more apprehensive about what was to come.

Especially welcome to Libby were visits by her inner circle of intimates, mostly women, who were escorts to her inner journey, her exploration of mortality, identity and meaning. Here I took a back seat. We all have our views but she needed a variety of ears and voices to guide her along the darkening path. She had told *The Times* she wanted 'a good death', like that of her sister and father, and seemed to have reached an almost clinical spirituality. I could only admire her grace but some-times, when confusion or anxiety was hitting her, I'd resort to blatant distractions. She'd mention a lump or a bleed, and I'd point to an early-flowering shrub or suggest a Jane Austen film, look out a Khalil Gibran poem or put on some Pergolesi. And then, out of the blue, she would suggest a meeting to fine-tune her funeral in Vowchurch or the Thanksgiving Service in London or to select the most environmentally responsible coffin. (For once, she wouldn't decide what to wear. I later chose a vivid red gown.) She could still laugh, and did, quite a lot.

Her lack of anger was astonishing. A strong woman of 65 strides across the Cevennes and within a week discovers she has a disease that is almost always fatal. But she has no anger at all with Fate or Chance or God? No complaint even, no trace of self-pity? She would only say that, having had her ovaries and breasts removed to avoid the cancer, she felt 'a bit miffed'.

She was still watching her body with close medical attention and found it fascinating. In the last week or two she became sure the end was close. She warned and comforted friends, stopped reading, closed her computer and told me she wanted no more questions about anything. Two afternoons before she died, Frances brought Communion to give us at the bedside but Libby continued to drowse. Frances gave it to me and then touched Libby's lips with a wafer dipped in the wine: Libby opened her eyes and quietly repeated the words of the service, twice over.

She spoke only once more, the day after. Having been told that hearing was the last sense to go, I whispered again that I was with her to the end, would always be with her. Her eyelids flickered and she said, 'Wonderful, wonderful.' The next evening, as Julia and I lay beside her on the bed, Julia whispered that she thought Libby had finally gone. We waited. No breathing. We wept.

Libby had enjoyed a highly successful career, written many books, helped thousands, made legions of friends worldwide and battled a cruel disease. But she hated attempts to make her a medical martyr or to thrust her on a pedestal. She thought such extravagant elevation laughable, not even decent. It was not that she 'believed in' self-effacement: she embodied it.

Did Libby have any faults? I tried to identify some, and asked her friends. They found it just as difficult as I to discover what, if any, faults Libby had. In the end the list hardly seems to count as faults at all. A bit controlling, yet often impulsive? Too particular? Sometimes too certain? Competitive? Somewhat head-girlish? More ambitious than she appeared? A fraction too unsuspicious of others' motives? A tad too nice? A bit too . . . uncomplicated?

(One paper had said her renowned enthusiasm was 'enervating', but they clearly meant stimulating.)

Yet is limitless 'can do' energy a fault when suffused with generosity? Can we disparage such devoted immersion in such valuable work or question her unalloyed joy in the beauties of nature, in being with friends? In simply being? Was her enthusiastic leadership and courage in adversity indebted to whatever had also enabled her war-hero and politician father to be a good leader – being strong, not tough, commanding through example, not dictation?

But I too totter on the cliff edge of idealisation, even heroine-worship. No wonder. Libby was far the best thing that ever happened to me. Her arrival in my life was like an act of Grace: unmerited, unaccountable, magical. Rachmaninov never mediated a more solid union. I wonder if it is normal to adore anyone so much. I looked it up today: adoration contains reverence. That fits. I revered her warmth and immediacy, her joy in life, her ready laughter, her steady realism, her simple courage, her spontaneous empathy with the distressed, her incandescent delight in friendship.

Surely few people have had so many: her friends queued to drive her across England for treatment. But the love that spilled so freely from her was not the product of virtue, effort or any coolly moral imperative. It was natural, as if compensation for her flawed genetic inheritance, another part of what she was. Her love was a natural phenomenon: spontaneous, flowing like sparkling water from an infinitely prolific spring. How lucky she and all of us have been!

Now her strange, cruel, beautiful and mysterious journey is over. As that prayer put it, the strife is over. There will be peace at last. I shall thank the heavens for her to my own dying day and we shall be together, always. I don't know whether we shall be put away in some retirement haven beyond the stars. That sort of thinking is unnecessary: we know what we mean.

For the funeral our old oak-framed church was filled with daffodils, crowded with people, many standing at the back. Felicity had crowned the plaited bamboo coffin with camellias, Faith gave a warmly affectionate tribute and Catrin played her harp and sang 'Singing the Life'. After the words 'Lord, now lettest thou thy servant depart in peace', Libby's four young nephews and nieces carried the coffin to her grave near some birch trees and we sang the hymns she had picked out as we threw Hereford's red soil into it.

Three days later I planted bulbs, laid wild daffodils at her feet and resolved to celebrate three wonderful decades with her, rather than lament the remaining one or two without her. Yet grief for so cruel and untimely a death needs no apology. It too calls out to be heard. And it too can strike us out of the blue or the dark. That sleepless night I listened to an opera new to me, Delibes's *Lakmé*. Suddenly there was a heart-piercing aria:

> *Beneath a star filled sky*
> *The dove has flown away.*
> *Come back, I am calling you.*
> *My sweet love, come back.*

Ronald Higgins
April, 2008

Appendix

Thoughts About BRCA1 and Some Other Inherited Diseases

BY 2006 THE mechanism of the BRCA1 gene was becoming better understood. It is now known that the job of the BRCA1 gene, together with BRCA2, is to prevent cells from growing and dividing too rapidly or in an uncontrolled way. BRCA1 provides instructions to a protein directly involved in the repair of damaged DNA. The gene probably interacts with many other proteins including other tumour suppressors and those that regulate the division of cells.

All cancers are genetic in that they arise from the action of genes, damaged ones. However, only 5–10 per cent of these damaged genes (mutations) are inherited from previous generations. In the other 90 per cent or so of cases the damage in the gene occurs in body cells during one's lifetime, a so-called 'acquired' mutation. The development of a cancer tumour involves a series of steps and it is as if at least one step has already occurred in those of us who carry an inherited mutation.

Genetic tests aim to identify gene mutations. The tests do not say whether or not an individual has or will develop cancer but they can clearly establish whether a mutation is present.

Overall, women who carry a BRCA1 mutation have an 80

per cent risk of developing cancer of the ovary or breast. If they develop breast cancer, unless they have a double mastectomy, there is a relatively high chance of one or more further tumours developing in the same or the other breast.

Whether BRCA1 and BRCA2 mutation carriers have an increased risk of cancers other than ovary and breast is uncertain. There does seem to be a slightly increased risk of cancer of the prostate, particularly in BRCA2 carriers. Studies on bowel and pancreatic cancer have not yet given a definite answer.

Cancer of the breast in men is extremely rare but is higher in BRCA1 and BRCA2 carriers than in the general population. For other cancers, particularly of the prostate, men with a BRCA2 mutation appear to carry a higher risk than those with a BRCA1 mutation. However in females the BRCA1 mutation is in general the more threatening.

What are the advantages of a woman knowing whether or not she has a BRCA1 mutation gene? Clearly if the test shows that she is not a carrier of the mutation, she can feel relieved and no longer needs special screening or to think about other measures such as removal of breasts and ovaries. Although the discovery that you are a carrier of the family cancer gene is bound to be unwelcome news, it does at least remove uncertainty and allows an informed choice about taking one or more of the various steps to reduce the risk before the cancer has had a chance to develop.

A positive BRCA1 test is upsetting but does not carry the devastating implications associated with, say, the inherited gene for Huntington's disease, which afflicts all who get it with a cruelly progressive mental and physical disorder.

Before the May 2006 decision, approval for PGD had largely been limited to hereditary disorders causing lifelong disability or death early in life, or to ones for which there was no treatment or means of prevention. PGD for cancer genes is much more controversial: not everyone who carries a BRCA1 mutation will develop cancer; preventive measures and treatment are available; and the cancer does not develop until later in life by which time there may well have been many new developments in its prevention, detection and treatment.

Following the announcement of the PGD option for BRCA1 carriers, I discussed the issues of genetic testing, preventive measures and PGD with a variety of people professionally involved. They included geneticists and genetic counsellors, practitioners in PGD, colleagues in counselling and psycho-therapy. I talked to a number of individuals who knew they had a hereditary cancer in their family and sent a confidential questionnaire to all my own first and second cousins or to their surviving partners.

Genetic Testing or Not?

The prime questions here are whether a given individual who knows herself or himself to be at risk should decide to have a test, if that is available, as for instance with BRCA1 and, if so, what they should do with the result. What also should be taken into account is whether or not information about genetic test results, and therefore of genetic risk, should be communicated to other members of the family and, if so, by whom.

Discussions on genetic testing too often lump all 'genetically testable' diseases together. But, apart from these diseases being very different in themselves, the implications of an abnormal gene can be very different. A disease such as cystic fibrosis will affect a child from birth and, for many, seriously reduce their quality of life.

Into another category come Huntington's disease and some others which can also be handed on to the next generation but allow a normal early life before causing its distressing and incurable mental and physical deterioration.

Yet another category consists of disorders which may vary greatly in how they express themselves, sometimes causing only minor signs and symptoms, if any at all, whereas in other people the effects may be seriously disabling or even life threatening.

BRCA1 cancer and other adult onset cancers come into a fourth category. Here, not only is the affected individual likely to have a normal life until middle age, but can take active steps to prevent the cancer developing or have it treated in its early stages. Furthermore many of these cancer genes do not invariably result in cancer in the carrier.

The questions to be considered before deciding on genetic testing would be different in the four categories. Not least of these considerations would be what actual difference the positive or negative finding could make either to the individual or to the family. Would the result allow measures to be taken that could prevent or at least, through early detection, successfully treat the disease?

Most people would consider the only justification for testing a child would be for conditions where the result could influence treatment during childhood. Otherwise the decision should surely be postponed until the individual becomes old enough to decide about testing for him or herself.

It is clear that many people do not want to know their

genetic status and will choose not to be tested even if they know they have as high as a 50/50 chance of carrying the affected gene. Others choose not to be tested because they fear the result may jeopardise their job opportunities, their chances of promotion or affect their health insurance. Some people choose to pay to have the test done by a commercial company on the web to avoid the results being included in their NHS records.[11]

Has an individual the right *not* to be tested? Do I have a right to remain in genetic ignorance? Many would argue that I do; that each of us has the right to decide for ourselves and that the new ability to test should not be translated into a moral compulsion. They would also say that refusal to be tested should be respected as a legitimate personal choice and not represented as a failure of courage. Others may say that I only have the right to ignorance if the test result concerns me alone and could not affect the health of other members of my family.

It is not only adults who have an incurable degenerative disease in the family who choose not to be tested. Some simply prefer to live in ignorance. Even those who may well be carriers of a gene for a potentially treatable disease, such as cancer, may prefer to avoid confirmation. Rather than have the genetic test, several members of my own family chose to have frequent and intense, yet possibly unnecessary, ovary and breast screening.

Some may be simply fearful of the possible result, preferring

---

[11] Many British citizens will be reassured by the decision in 2005 by the UK Government and the Association of British Insurers to extend the voluntary moratorium on the use of predictive genetic results by insurers until 2011. This confirms that genetic tests cannot be used to deny insurance cover – for the time being anyway.

to do nothing. Others who say they will let 'fate' decide, may then feel subsequent guilt if they develop cancer, pass the cancer gene on to their child, or both.

Genetic testing resolves uncertainty for those who are found to be free of the gene mutation but those who find they are indeed cancer gene carriers may well suffer a lonely anxiety wondering whether, when and where the disease may hit. It could be in a few months or it could be decades. Or they might be one of the lucky 20 per cent who never develop the disease. Being at risk means feeling different from those who do not carry the gene, or brothers who may transmit it, and also from those who have already developed cancer. It is an emotionally ambiguous state on its own and could involve fear, anxiety, envy, hostility or excessive dependency.

Imposing possibly upsetting or unwanted information on the younger generation clearly requires careful thought. A parent or grandparent may feel he or she is doing their children a service by being tested even if the result will not be of any practical consequence for the individual in question. However, the result will inevitably affect the children's chances or, more accurately, their *perceived* chances, for better or worse, of being a cancer gene carrier. If any individual chooses to be tested for the BRCA1 mutation the perceived odds of their siblings, children and grandchildren carrying the cancer gene will change. In reality of course an individual either 100 per cent carries the gene mutation or is 100 per cent free from it. If he or she is found *not* to carry the mutation then their children and grandchildren must be clear of it too. If it is found they do carry the mutation their children's chance of carrying it increases to 50 per cent. Many people would find living with a 50 per cent risk very different to living with a 12.5 per cent let alone a 6.25 per cent risk which is the position of some of the members of the youngest generation in our extended family. Many would therefore feel that adult children should be consulted before a parent arranges to be tested.

On the other hand others may consider it their parental duty to be tested and to tell their children the results when they feel they're at a suitable age, whether positive or negative. In our own family, however, some of the older members of our wider family, already themselves beyond the high-risk stage of developing cancer, decided not to be tested. They believed that it was for their children themselves to decide whether they wanted to be tested.

Some of my own generation didn't even know there was such a test available for our cancer gene. Others had decided against it on grounds of cost or because they thought it would affect their own or their children's financial circumstances. In the UK and in Canada testing is free of charge, although one male relative in the UK was quite erroneously told by their doctor that the test was unnecessary in males. In America the test would currently cost something over $300 and about the same in South Africa. In addition there will often be considerable expenses in travelling, say, to one of the only three genetics units in South Africa that can provide the necessary testing and the mandatory genetic counselling that precedes and follows it.

Two older members of our own family felt that much unnecessary anxiety might be relieved if they were tested and found to be negative. This proved to be the case with my father's sister who was tested in her late eighties. Her negative finding meant that her 14 descendants over three generations were all cleared. Of course it could also be argued that had she turned out to be one of the 20 per cent of carriers who do not develop cancer despite a long life, the family's anxiety would have been greatly increased. Nevertheless, knowing that their mother or grandmother was a carrier, would at least have allowed each descendant to make an informed choice as to the test and, if necessary, to preventive measures.

Among the many family members of my own generation there was wide variation in the amount of information and encouragement in relation to genetic testing that they were giving to the next generation (most now with children themselves). Even though all but one of the surviving parents knew of the family cancer, some had not told their older children. Others had discussed it in a non-directive way. Still others had actively, even persistently, encouraged their children to be tested.

Of course even those who test negative carry some risk of cancer, the same risk as that of anyone in the general population. Not surprisingly women who have been elated to learn they are not carrying their family's cancer gene may be especially devastated if they go on to develop a non-inherited breast cancer.

For some families the waiting for their own family's gene mutation to be identified can be very stressful. One 40-year-old with an affected mother and aunt had reluctantly decided she would have both her ovaries and breasts removed if she knew *for certain* that she too carried the cancer gene. After three years of research their family's specific cancer gene mutation has yet to be discovered. The geneticist is hopeful that 'it will not be long'. How long can she afford to wait? Meanwhile her own mother, having suffered from cancer herself and watched her sister do so, is anxious that her daughter should not delay her preventive surgery.

Such pressures and prolonged uncertainties can greatly add to the overall distress of families who may well already be suffering from bereavement and recurrent life-threatening illnesses. Even for those with a strong family history of cancer, the final confirmation of a gene mutation can be tough:

> I got my genetic results last week and I have BRCA2, which I suppose was a bit of a shock, but after all I did want to know and perhaps it is a relief, even though it means alerting quite a few members of the family.

Others, with a strong family history of cancer, may have lived with the assumption that they too were carriers of the cancer gene and feel the test is unnecessary:

> I always thought I would get breast cancer and the test would have confirmed my thoughts, and I would not have decided (I don't think) to have a double mastectomy on the results of the blood test. . . Having had a mastectomy [for breast cancer] I still declined a double mastectomy – maybe I'm just a born optimist!

Genetic diseases, whether BRCA1 or others, that are known to run within a family can have divisive and emotionally devastating effects on relationships. One mother shared with me her distress over the impossibility of catering for her own wishes, yet also the needs of her ex husband – the carrier of the abnormal gene in this case – their son and his new partner:

He didn't want me to investigate, while I wanted to know. His reasons were that he wanted our son to live a carefree life, as he had done, and face the problem just when it arose. I wanted to know, but was very torn. Was it my right to investigate a disease? . . . Was I tormenting my son with my wish to know?

The father's insistence on concealment meant that the son did not know that he could himself be a carrier and, if so, that there would be measures he could be taking at least to delay the onset of the disease. And the son in turn was unwittingly concealing vital information from his new partner, not only about his own life-threatening disease but about one that could be inherited by any children they might have.

Preventive Measures or Not?

It was clear that many people felt there were ethical issues concerning genetic testing for BRCA1 but that these did not on the whole apply to the use of preventive measures like screening or surgery. There were certainly differences of opinion as to how far to go but these did not appear to be based on questions of right and wrong. The decisions were usually being made pragmatically – on the perceived balance between the negatives and positives. A greatly reduced risk of developing breast or ovarian cancer had to be weighed against the possible pain, disfigurement and other side effects of surgery as well as often many years of replacement hormones. The equation can of course vary greatly with different individuals and with changing circumstances, as it did in my own case.

One colleague wrote of a client:

She has had three or four cancerous breast lumps removed, I think all primaries. She was recently advised to have her ovaries removed post-haste and has done so. I asked her why she does not have a mastectomy, and she says she thinks that if the cancer develops in her breasts, at least it can be dealt with. If she has them removed, she believes the cancer might develop elsewhere where it is less accessible.

When cancer appeared in my pancreas, I tried to resist asking myself whether I might have been better off if I had not had my breasts removed. I did not always succeed.

Some who had planned to have preventive surgery may be disconcerted, or even change their minds, when they learn that the risks of ovarian or breast cancer cannot be entirely eliminated. Following the removal of the ovaries there is still a small risk of cancer developing in the membranes lining the abdomen, the peritoneum. And with the breasts a tiny piece of vulnerable tissue may remain despite extensive surgery.

As surgical techniques advance, an increasing number of surgeons and potential cancer victims are prepared to consider major surgery. In November 2006 two sisters in their early twenties were reported as having their stomachs removed on the same day because they were known to carry a defective gene that had caused fatal stomach cancer in their father, cousin and grandmother (*Sunday Times*, 12 November 2006). A family of three sisters with the BRCA2 mutation all had double mastectomies within a few months of each other (*Daily Telegraph*, 4 October 2006).

Reaching a decision about major surgery can be a prolonged, complicated and painful process:

My parents had been urging me to do so for years when it became clear I was not going to have children. I eventually and reluctantly promised my father before he died that I would have the op [removal of the ovaries] and then experienced a huge amount of internal turmoil over whether to do it or not. Eventually the uncertainty got to me to such an extent that I booked the operation. . .

However I was so ambivalent about the whole thing (I hate the concept of removing healthy organs) that I told [the Research Centre] that they could have my tissue and that they had my permission to examine it but that I did not want to know whether or not I was carrying the gene. I still don't know. . .

Both in relation to genetic testing and surgery, there were some who were fatalistic and felt that whatever shall be, should be. Others did not want to think about it or repeatedly said they intended to take some action but kept putting it off.

Pre-implantation Genetic Diagnosis or Not?
Not surprisingly none of our family members had yet used PGD for BRCA1 or for any other reason, or indeed had had cause to consider it for themselves. Only one had even heard of it in relation to BRCA1.

There is no doubt that PGD with embryo selection raises far more ethical dilemmas than any other issues faced by families with a BRCA1 cancer gene. It is an area in which I have been interested for many years. Not only had I been one of the inspectors of fertility clinics for the Human Fertilisation and Embryology Authority but I had also counselled couples facing the agonising dilemma of whether their recently conceived triplet (or more) pregnancy should best be reduced by surgical intervention to two fetuses, or even one – the so called multi-fetal pregnancy reduction. The idea of effectively creating embryos through artificial means and then destroying one or more of the resulting fetuses can be distressing to anyone and completely unacceptable to some.

Embryo selection following PGD is not the same as multi-fetal pregnancy reduction in that the embryos that are discarded in PGD will never have been implanted in the womb, so a pregnancy has not been established. Nevertheless, both procedures can be seen by some people as the destruction of a potential fetus, a potential child. Others feel that it is interfering to an unacceptable degree with what they see as Nature or the Will of God. Some claim that conception should only result from the natural act of sexual intercourse.

Most of the people I contacted, including some counsellors, had not heard of PGD for BRCA1 and so were unable to offer an informed or fully considered opinion.

Within one of my cousins' families two sisters had very different views from fully supportive to:

> I feel that nature must to a certain extent be allowed to run her course. If there are tests available now, for diagnosing and treating cancers, in the future they will be even better. To start deciding which embryo will be implanted or not I feel is interfering too much. I also have slight concerns about long-term effects of mass production of selection of embryos for all types of potential or future problems, not just familial cancers. Will there be no normal pregnancies?

But she went on to emphasise:

> The final decision is with the parents and they need to be supported in their decision. Parents should be able to decide what they are capable of handling and living with. . . It is difficult to refuse a foetus a chance of being born if the disease threatening him or her is treatable.

I have to recognise that, had our own parents used PGD, neither I nor my two sisters would have existed. They would probably have had three children but they wouldn't have been us. However I don't believe this idea is a useful contribution to the argument for or against PGD. It is just a fact that cannot be escaped and one that many people put to me, and some find powerful.

One relative who on religious grounds would not consider PGD wrote:

> I do not think genetic engineering is appropriate in this case. It is a theological question: what is the purpose of human life? While it is natural for us all to desire a 'long and happy one' that is not the purpose of our existence. Christian theology understands our purpose in relation to God our Creator. The purpose of life on this earth is to grow in our relationship with God, and to serve and praise Him in the way we live, with confidence in His loving care for us in all eternity. On earth we live imperfect lives in an imperfect world. I understand the role of medical science to be to relieve suffering and to combat disease. It is not its role to create a superhuman race by removing all conceived deficiencies from the gene pool.

Of course PGD does not involve 'genetic engineering' as no gene is altered by the procedure but this unfortunately remains a common misconception.

However, not all religious perspectives lead to the same conclusion. Several Anglican priests with whom I spoke, while finding the procedure distressing, did not find it theologically unacceptable. On the other hand some people with no religious belief, nevertheless found the procedure totally unacceptable. One agnostic friend who knows herself to be at risk of a familial cancer was strongly against PGD. She told me:

My reasons are that cancer research is moving so fast that the probability of new preventative medicine in the future is very great. Also if I had the cancer ones removed and then gave birth to a Down's syndrome or an autistic child I would kick myself for meddling with nature.

She later wrote:

I have been thinking about deleting embryos with the cancer gene. I am more and more and more against it. . . We would not have had you. Whatever happens you have had a good 60 odd years, done a lot for the planet, and brought great joy. Appalling that anyone could think they can act God and delete [cancer gene carrying] embryos. I am getting quite angry about it as I write. Having said all that, there are some embryos that I would delete. Those that would definitely have no quality of life from day one. I wish people would stop making all these decisions possible. . .

Cancer seems to me to be a lot better than most things in that one can have a very, very fulfilling life until it strikes, which is usually not until middle age. Think what great men have died in their thirties and left great works. Many many artists.

A child who carries the BRCA1 mutation is no less, or more, likely than any other child to suffer from an additional abnormality such as Down's syndrome. However, several people felt, however illogically, that PGD was somehow tempting fate.

The views of one doctor specialising in research on the BRCA1 gene, were representative of a number of his colleagues. Although he was not against PGD for conditions which seriously affected the young child, he felt that in diseases that only had an onset in adulthood, decisions had to be made by the person themselves and could not be taken by a parent. Thus, for him, PGD for BRCA1 should not be an option. Weight was added to his view by the fact that a significant percentage – 20 per cent – of gene carriers would never develop cancer at all and far more would not die from it either because of preventive surgery or early detection and treatment.

A different view was expressed by one counsellor:

I don't expect cancer to make any sense to me, I don't feel suffering has a purpose, I think if the suffering, grief and devastation of early death can be avoided, (there is enough around that is still completely beyond any control) then we should use the knowledge now available to do so (i.e. PGD and embryo selection).

A psychiatrist experienced in talking to couples considering PGD wrote:

The fact is that still healthy carriers consider even pre-implantation diagnosis like a cruel selection and a personal wound. The whole question stirs up all sorts of largely unconscious fears of being unwanted, rejected, considered defective or a second-class human being. . . I have seen many prospective parents reacting like this especially when the genetic disease had not yet manifested itself. Pre-implantation embryo selection. . . was equated with abortion, and furthermore the identification with the discarded embryo or fetus [can be] too strong. In my experience it is very difficult to disentangle these issues. . . many carriers I counselled in the end preferred not to know and not to choose.

What is very clear, and has been shown repeatedly, is that for most people the concept of PGD and embryo selection is new and, for many, baffling. Few psychotherapists and counsellors will have met couples who have had PGD and there is still much to learn about the emotional implications. Although there are excellent genetic counsellors available, even these are often faced with new situations such as a young couple, one of whom is a BRCA1 carrier.

One of the basic difficulties for such worried couples is their lack of personal experience. The woman carrier is unlikely herself to have suffered from cancer before she is planning her first pregnancy although she may have witnessed the suffering of her mother. A male carrier may have to confide in a female partner who has had no experience of cancer in either a close relative or friend. As one counsellor wrote:

There is something very different about BRCA1 and other later developing genetically determined diseases. This is not about living with a disability, about living a life from the beginning with the disease. But it *is* about living with the possibility of untimely death, about people living with the loss of parents at an early age, about waiting for cancer to strike.

However, even in the case of a lifelong disabling disease, such as the dominantly inherited Brittle Bone Disease (osteogenesis imperfecta), mothers' views on embryo selection can differ. One woman may say she does not want to put her child through what she's been through, whereas another may feel she has had a rich and full life despite the disease. Inevitably their perceptions of their own experiences will colour their attitudes towards PGD.

By the end of 2006 only one fertility unit in the UK had actually applied to test for BRCA1 by PGD but several were considering doing so. Currently a unit wishing to perform PGD on a BRCA1 or 2 carrier would need to apply for permission for each individual case. In the past, relatively few couples have gone to the lengths of having PGD even with life-threatening diseases. It seems likely that fewer still will take advantage of this option for a BRCA1 mutation. The PGD/IVF procedure is inevitably stressful both physically and psychologically. Moreover the pregnancy success rate following IVF is currently only one in five attempts (although it could well prove higher for these couples who have no infertility problems as such). Couples may also be concerned that the PGD procedure itself might be harmful to their child. Although initial studies show no evidence that the interference with the embryo in PGD causes any long-term damage, inevitably these studies need to be on larger numbers and for many more years before couples (and their doctors) can feel completely reassured.

Another discouragement is that the whole procedure is likely to prove expensive. Although the testing of the embryo for the gene mutation through PGD may be available free on the NHS, many couples would find themselves having to pay for one, two or sometimes many more IVF procedures, each costing several thousand pounds. This would be especially galling for normally fertile couples who could otherwise have expected to become pregnant through natural means – and free of charge. Such couples would also of course need to practise birth control. There are clearly big, often daunting, decisions for a young couple to make, especially when the concepts involved are likely to be new to at least one of the partners.

Readers may be surprised that I have not said how I stand myself on the option of PGD. One reason has been that I have wanted to explore without prejudice the many positions professionals among others have been taking on this relatively new and certainly complex issue. Perhaps most of all I do not wish to risk swaying the decisions yet to be made by my nieces and nephews but rather to help them to understand and carefully weigh the wide range of views and the options available to them – and in due course their partners.

Glossary

Allele

One of two or more alternative forms of a gene at a given position (locus) on a chromosome. It is one of a series of DNA codes that are useful to determine whether or not a disease is shared by members of the same family.

Autosome

Any chromosome other than a sex chromosome. Humans have 22 pairs of autosomes.

BRCA1/BRCA2

BRCA1/BRCA2 are tumour suppressor genes that are important for the repair of damaged DNA. If a person inherits certain altered versions (mutations) of the gene, they have a high risk of developing breast and ovarian cancer.

Carrier

An individual who does not necessarily manifest a condition but who carries a gene for it and can therefore pass this gene on to offspring who may under certain circumstances exhibit the condition.

Glossary

Chromosome

A rod-shaped body made of DNA found in the nucleus of every cell in the body. Chromosomes carry the genes that determine the characteristics of an individual.

Humans have 23 pairs of chromosomes in each cell – 22 pairs of autosomes and one pair of sex chromosomes. Each parent contributes one chromosome to each pair, so children get half of their chromosomes from their mothers and half from their fathers.

Chromosome 17q

The long arm (q) of the 17th chromosome where the BRCA1 gene is positioned. A mutation due to deletion of a segment of this chromosome may cause ovarian or breast cancer.

DNA (deoxyribonucleic acid)

DNA is the material of which genes are composed. A DNA molecule is made up of four units (called bases) that are designated A, T, G and C [see *Genetic code* below]. The sequence of the bases spell out instructions for making all of the proteins in an organism. A change in one of the DNA letters making up a gene is a mutation. In some cases, these mutations can alter the protein instructions and lead to disease. Each individual passes their chromosomes on to their children, and therefore pass down the DNA instructions.

Dominant inheritance

The type of inheritance in which only one of the pair of chromosomes needs to carry the affected gene for an individual to manifest the trait (e.g. cancer). If a condition is inherited dominantly, it can be passed on from an affected parent to an offspring, even though the other parent does not carry the gene for the disease. Each time an affected person has a child, there is a 50/50 chance that the child will be affected.

Embryo selection

The choice of one or more embryos that have been tested by PGD to be free from a particular genetic abnormality before transfer to the womb.

Familial

A condition that 'runs in the family'.

First-degree relative

A relative who is one step away along the family tree – parent, full sibling or child.

Gene

The basic unit of heredity. Genes are arranged along chromosomes in the centre of each cell. They are made up of DNA. The precise sequence of the DNA determines the precise nature of the protein for which the gene codes for a particular characteristic or function.

Genetic code

The instructions in a gene that tell the cell how to make a specific protein. A, T, G and C are the 'letters' of the DNA code; they stand for the chemicals adenine, thymine, guanine and cytosine, that make up the nucleotide bases of DNA. Each gene's code combines the four chemicals in various ways to spell out three-letter 'words' that specify which amino acid is needed at every step in making a protein.

Genetic counselling

A short-term educational counselling process for individuals and families who have a genetic disease or who are at risk from such a disease. Genetic counselling provides patients with information about their condition and helps them make informed decisions.

Genotype

The genetic constitution of an individual. The total of all the genes carried by that person, whether expressed or not.

Germline mutation

– see **Hereditary mutation** below.

Haplotype

A haplotype is what makes up, genetically, each individual chromosome. It is used to ascertain whether or not a disease has genetic origins.

Hereditary

Transmission from parent to child of information contained in the genes.

Hereditary mutation

A gene change in the body's reproductive cells (egg or sperm) that becomes incorporated into the DNA of every cell in the body of offspring; hereditary mutations are passed on from parents to offspring.

Hysterectomy
Removal of the womb.

In vitro fertilisation
Fertilisation of the egg outside the woman's body. This may be done in cases of infertility or to enable pre-implantation genetic diagnosis to be done.

Inherited
Transmission of a trait through genes from parents to offspring.

Karyotype
An individual's full chromosome complement.

Mastectomy
Removal of the breast.

Maternal
On the mother's side.

Mutation
A permanent structural alteration in DNA. These alterations can cause or predispose an individual to a specific disease.

Oophorectomy
Removal of the ovary.

Glossary

Paternal
On the father's side.

Pre-implantation genetic diagnosis (PGD)
The use of reproductive technology (IVF and embryo biopsy) together with genetic techniques to identify unaffected embryos for implantation in the womb.

Prophylactic oophorectomy
Removal of healthy ovaries in order to reduce the risk of disease.

Recessive inheritance
A condition that is only manifest if copies of the relevant gene code are present in both of a pair of chromosomes. The condition can only occur when both parents carry a gene for the disorder.

Second-degree relative
A relative who is two steps away along the family tree – grandparents, grandchildren, aunts, uncles, nephews and nieces.

Serum CA-125
A blood test that measures the level of CA-125, a substance found in blood, other body fluids and some tissues. Increased levels of CA-125 may be a sign of ovarian cancer.

Tumour suppressor gene
A protective gene that normally limits the growth of tumours. When a tumour suppressor gene is mutated, it may fail to prevent a cancer from growing. BRCA1 and BRCA2 are tumour suppressor genes.

Acknowledgements

THE WHOLE BOOK is an expression of gratitude to all my family, friends and colleagues who have travelled with me through these last two years. Only a few are mentioned by name in the book. I want therefore to acknowledge some others who have been especially involved either in producing the book or in giving me the strength to write it.

But there are even more friends who remain unnamed. I trust they realise how grateful I am for their cherishing during the dark days – each one who visited, sent a card, a letter, an email, a book, flowers, chocolate, cakes, chicken soup and other freezer fillers or yet more eccentric gifts. Many generously held me in their thoughts or prayers.

Some of our neighbours gave invaluable practical help and friendship week after week: Frances Lewis, Guama Mathai, Rex and Eva Morris, Brian and Sylvia Price.

For many years I have appreciated Jane Gardiner's help with my medical work but the generous gift of her time to help with our regular newsletters went far beyond the call of duty.

Yorkshire friends and others from my childhood became a special source of support, not least Rosemary and Anthony

Acknowledgements

Preston (whose home, car and friendship were always so generously given). My chemotherapy ordeal was greatly eased by visitors who sometimes travelled many miles to share my regular picnic lunch in the Cancer Clinic. They included Eileen Aris, Ilona Bendefy, Christine and Peter Burton, Frances Hancock, Maggie Linford, Daniel and Barbara McDowell, Marilyn Pietroni, Hermione Raven, Sue Sabbagh and Jonathan Stedall.

I thank my friends in the Multiple Births Foundation, the Twins and Multiple Births Association, Multiple Births Canada and the International Society for Twin Studies for persisting through this time in keeping me in touch with the world of twins. I thank also my many friends in Home Start.

Tribute is due to the three people without whom my career in paediatrics and later interest in multiple births could never have blossomed – Pamela Davies, David Harvey and the late Walter Henderson.

My recovery was hastened by the restorative welcome of so many Australian friends, like Christine Johnston and Steve and Sue Baddeley whose apartments in Melbourne and Sydney became our havens. And later by friends at the Champernowne Trust week such as Andy Clements and Mike Vizard and by the 'Monmouth team' who welcomed us back for the annual walk on the continent despite my faltering steps.

Sue Norrington, Anne Ashley Cooper and the late Clare Brennan provided inspiration and humour that only fellow travellers could give.

I have throughout had most helpful discussions in Cambridge with Professsor Bruce Ponder at the Cancer Research Unit and also with Carole Pye, Professor Martin

Richards of the Family Research Centre and Dr Andrew Tutt of Breakthrough. I am grateful to Mr Darius Mirza, my surgeon, Dr Richard Griffiths, my GP, and Professor Patrick Pietroni for checking some medical aspects and to Patrick for his thoughtful and thought-provoking contribution to Chapter 17.

Colleagues and friends who have contributed or commented on the psychological and ethical issues include Jenny Clifford, Jean Curtis Raleigh, Jane Denton, Peter Dunn, Lynette Findlay, Alison Lashwood, Vivienne Lewin, Pam Mills, Lalage Neal, Sue Norrington, Fiona Palmer Barnes, Alessandra Piontelli, Sue Ramsbotham, Barbara Read, Carrie Rowell, Richard Rowson, Meriel Tegner, Julia Waite and Clare Ziegler.

If there are factual errors or misjudgements the responsibility is however entirely mine.

Ron and Hilary Nicholls provided invaluable information on our family tree and my friend and neighbour Cynthia Comyn, who works at the College of Arms, is responsible for the beautiful genealogy chart. Marion Paterson of the Multiple Births Foundation kindly helped me with the design of some of the figures.

The title had many versions. I thank Theo Richmond and Lee Langley for many of the more interesting ones and for their ongoing enthusiasm in the search. For permission to reproduce the song 'I Sing the Life' from which the title is derived I thank the author, Jane Mayers.

My debt to Julia Gregson is huge. Not only did she inspire me to start the book, but loyally read each chapter, encouraging me through the lows and blocks and offering valuable ideas with such tact that I was tempted to think them my own.

I will not again mention all the many members of my

Acknowledgements

extended family to whom I am indebted except Norman Macrae, Heather Craig and Nancy Maguire, my father's first cousins, who put me in touch with all my own and younger generations; my stepmother Cynthia Bryan for permission to quote from my father's published writings; my brother-in-law Rob Hingley for permission to quote extensively from my late sister Bernadette Hingley's unpublished writings; my niece Liz Hingley for her photographs; my niece Catherine Hingley for her written contribution and two poems; my sister Felicity Bryan for her own written contributions and for permission to quote from her late daughter, Alice Duncan's, writing and, most of all, for her sisterly encouragement and professional advice on the whole manuscript.

My editors at Random House, Clare Hulton and Imogen Fortes, have given constant encouragement and many constructive suggestions. I also thank my publicist Emma Dowson.

It is difficult adequately to thank my literary agent, Carol Heaton. Rarely can one have been asked to combine such extensive professional guidance with such a close and supportive friendship. This she did with a sensitivity and generosity for which I am profoundly grateful. I also thank the whole team at Greene & Heaton for their help and warm encouragement, and especially Will Francis for some inspired suggestions.

And finally I must of course thank my husband Ronald Higgins for his written contributions and editorial improvements but incomparably more for continuing to travel patiently and lovingly with me through every stage of this long and bumpy journey. There have been tears but also much laughter in what in some ways have been the best two of our 29 years together.